TERENCE KEALEY trained in medicine at Barts Hospital Medical School, University of London (1970–76) ahead of moving to Oxford for a PhD in clinical biochemistry. From Oxford he moved to the University of Newcastle before, via a Wellcome Senior Clinical Research Fellowship, lecturing in clinical biochemistry at Cambridge (1986–2001). Between 2001 and 2014 he was Vice Chancellor of the University of Buckingham, and he is now a visiting scholar at the Center for the Study of Science at the Cato Institute, Washington, DC, where he is focusing on food policy.

Breakfast is a Dangerous Meal

WHY YOU SHOULD DITCH YOUR MORNING
MEAL FOR HEALTH AND WELLBEING

Terence Kealey

4th ESTATE • *London*

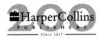

4th Estate
An imprint of HarperCollins*Publishers*
1 London Bridge Street
London SE1 9GF
www.4thEstate.co.uk

First published in Great Britain by 4th Estate in 2016

1 3 5 7 9 8 6 4 2

Copyright © Terence Kealey 2016

The right of Terence Kealey to be identified as the author
of this work has been asserted by him in accordance
with the Copyright, Design and Patents Act 1988

A catalogue record for this book is available from the British Library

ISBN 978-0-00-817234-3

Diagrams redrawn by Martin Brown

Typeset in Sabon and Helvetica Neue by Birdy Book Design

Printed and bound in Great Britain by Clays Ltd, St Ives plc

MIX
Paper from
responsible sources
FSC™ C007454

FSC™ is a non-profit international organisation established to promote
the responsible management of the world's forests. Products carrying the
FSC label are independently certified to assure consumers that they come
from forests that are managed to meet the social, economic and
ecological needs of present and future generations,
and other controlled sources.

Find out more about HarperCollins and the environment at
www.harpercollins.co.uk/green

To my wife, Sally

Contents

Prologue

I was contracted to submit the first draft of this manuscript to my publishers on 31 January 2016. The day before, on 30 January, *The Times* trailed on its front page an article by Angela Epstein, a health journalist, entitled 'Eight great weight-loss myths'. Skipping breakfast was myth number four:

> A recent study by Louisiana State University found that a 250-calorie serving of oatmeal [porridge] for breakfast resulted in reduced calorie intake at lunch.

Some people like to do the crossword, but my morning hobby is to find the catch in claims that breakfast is good for me, so where was this article's catch? I had twenty-four hours in which to uncover it.

It wasn't hard to locate the study, which had just been published in the *Journal of the American College of Nutrition*, where I discovered that it had actually come jointly from Louisiana State University and PepsiCo (which owns the Quaker Oats Company).[1] That is obviously a different provenance than from Louisiana State University alone.

The study showed, moreover, that, compared with a breakfast of Honey Nut Cheerios, a bowl of Quaker Instant Oatmeal slightly reduced the amount eaten subsequently at lunch; but the study did not compare subjects who ate a bowl of Quaker Instant Oatmeal with those who'd actually skipped breakfast, because no subjects were asked to skip it. Why not?

Well, it so happens that, contrary to what most people believe, eating breakfast significantly increases your total intake of calories: though eating breakfast may reduce your calorie intake at lunch, the calories you consume at breakfast will greatly exceed the ones they displace at lunch. So a fuller *Times* report of the study in the *Journal of the American College of Nutrition* might have read:

> A recent study by Louisiana State University that was funded by – and performed jointly with – PepsiCo (which owns the Quaker Oats Company) found that a 250-calorie serving of oatmeal for breakfast resulted in a slightly reduced calorie intake at lunch compared with an equivalent serving of Honey Nut Cheerios. Eating any cereal, however, greatly increases the total daily calorie intake, and only if breakfast were actually skipped would the total calorie intake have fallen.

That little story summarises this book.

Preface

Every morning Providence provides us with a precious gift, the gift of fasting. Overnight we digest the food we've eaten the day before, and by morning our metabolism has transitioned from feeding to fasting mode.

Fasting is a wonderfully healthy state. When we fast, our insulin levels fall, as do our blood sugar, triglyceride and cholesterol levels. Most usefully, when we fast, we lose weight. But what do too many of us do on waking? We break that lovely gift of fasting – we literally breakfast – and we eat, so courting type 2 diabetes, obesity, heart disease, strokes, hypertension, dementia and cancers of the liver, breast, pancreas and uterus.

Breakfast damages us in at least four different ways. First, it increases (not decreases) the number of calories we consume. Second, it provokes hunger pangs later in the day. Third, it aggravates the metabolic syndrome, which is the mass killer of our day, which – fourth – is further aggravated by the fact that breakfast is generally a carbohydrate-laden meal.

Breakfast may be the most important meal of the day, but only if we skip it.

PART ONE

My Story, Episode 1

How I discovered that breakfast is dangerous

1

My diagnosis

On 24 May 2010 my wife drove me to our family doctor's surgery and told me not to emerge without a diagnosis. Over the previous two or so months I had started to feel increasingly thirsty, and I had not only started to drink water all day but I had also started to pee all day. And all night. I was losing weight, my muscles were wasting away with a strange 'crackling' ache, and I felt tired all the time. I even woke in the morning feeling tired. Clearly, my wife said, I had developed diabetes, and she was irritated by my assurances that if we ignored the symptoms they might go away. So it was she who made the appointment to see our doctor, and it was she who drove us to the surgery to ensure I kept it.

I told my doctor what was happening and, echoing my wife, he said it sounded a bit like diabetes. I was forced to agree. So he performed a spot urine test, and there it was – glucose in my urine ('sugar in the water,' as he put it). I was diabetic. He then sent a blood sample to the lab, which shortly revealed a fasting blood glucose level of 19.3 mmol/l (normal range 3.9 to 5.5) and an HbA1c of 13.3 per cent (normal range 4 to 5.9; see later). I was very diabetic indeed. Type 2.

My story should thereafter have been routine. Thanks to a good wife and a good doctor a correct diagnosis had been made, and I was surely on the road to recovery. But I was then told to eat breakfast.

The authorities: Diabetes UK is the major diabetic charity in Britain. It was founded in 1934 as the Diabetic Association by H.G. Wells, the author, and by Dr R.D. Lawrence, a prominent physician, both of whom were diabetic. In 2013 its membership exceeded 300,000 people and its income was £38.8 million.[1] It is universally respected, both for its research and for its support for patients. Here is some dietary advice from its *Eating Well With Type 2 Diabetes*:

> **Eat three meals a day** [in bold in the publication]. Avoid skipping meals and space out your breakfast, lunch and evening meal over the day. This will not only help control your appetite but will also help control your blood glucose levels.[2]

And in case we don't get the message, Diabetes UK and the NHS have combined to reiterate, in red in the joint publication:

> **Don't skip breakfast.**[3]

The American Diabetes Association (ADA) is another impressive body. It has a membership of 441,000 and an annual turnover of $222 million,[4] and it recommends an even more generous frequency of eating, suggesting that diabetics eat: 'breakfast, lunch, dinner, and two snacks'.[5]

The diabetic charities certainly believe in frequent meals, and equally they believe in breakfast. So when, on diagnosing my diabetes, my doctor recommended I eat three meals a day including breakfast – as well as frequent snacks – he was only following the internationally agreed guidelines.

My glucometer: I might never have discovered how bizarre was that advice and those guidelines if our family doctor hadn't also given me a personal glucose meter or glucometer. This is a hand-held device, not much larger than a mobile phone, that allows people to monitor their fingerprick blood glucose levels several times a day. Because it provides the patient with direct access to the mysteries of their own disease, the glucometer is the diabetic equivalent of the ninety-five theses Martin Luther reportedly hammered into the church door in Wittenberg: it allows the patient to bypass the doctor, the NHS and the diabetes charities as directly as Luther once bypassed the pope, so patients can test the official advice against their own blood glucose levels.

On using my glucometer I soon made an unexpected discovery. I found that my blood glucose levels were dismayingly high first thing in the morning, but – even worse – they would rise much further, indeed hazardously, if I ate breakfast. I didn't feel ill with those elevated levels (glucose in high concentrations is a silent killer), but over time they would be killing me.

Yet if I skipped breakfast, my blood glucose levels would fall to normal over the morning. After lunch and dinner, of course, they would rise again, but noticeably less than after breakfast. Since high blood glucose levels are unsafe, I had discovered that, as a type 2 diabetic, breakfast was the most dangerous meal of my day. On reviewing the research journals, moreover, I found I hadn't been the first person to make that discovery. One of the pioneers was Professor Jens Christiansen from the department of medicine at the University of Aarhus in Denmark.

Professor Christiansen's experiment: Figure 1.1 shows the typical twenty-four-hour blood glucose profile of a group of healthy young people who eat three meals a day.[6]

As you can see, blood glucose levels between meals normally run at around 4–5 mmol/l. Within an hour of eating, however, those levels rise to well over 6. Yet within six hours of eating, those levels fall back to around 4–5.*

To see what happens in type 2 diabetes, Professor Christiansen and his colleagues monitored the blood glucose levels

---

* In the diabetic community, the words 'glucose' and 'sugar' are often used interchangeably. Glucose is in fact only one of many sugars, yet it is the most important of the blood and urine sugars, so the two terms are often interchanged.

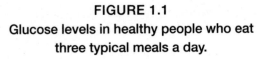

FIGURE 1.1
Glucose levels in healthy people who eat
three typical meals a day.

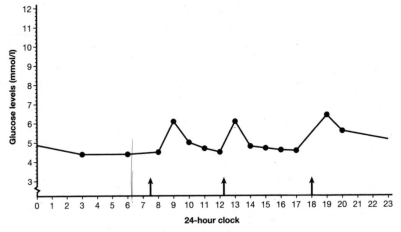

21 healthy subjects eating typical meals were studied and their results
averaged. The arrows indicate that breakfast was served at 7.30, lunch at
12.15 and dinner at 18.00. The results are from interstitial fluid,
which is similar to blood plasma and serum.

of thirteen adult patients. On some days he asked his thirteen
patients to skip breakfast, whereas on others he asked them to
eat it. To ensure that all other conditions were unchanged, he
asked his patients on breakfast-free days to compensate by eating more for lunch and dinner, so their daily energy intake was
the same. Figure 1.2A shows his patients' blood glucose levels
on the days they ate breakfast.[7]

As you can see, these diabetics start their days in a hazardous
state: their overnight fasting blood glucose levels are not much
short of 7.0 mmol/l. But look what happens after breakfast.
When patients are fed a full breakfast of about 600 calories
(between a quarter and a third of a day's intake of energy) their
blood glucose levels spike at around 10.5. These come down
within four hours, but that spike will have done the patients no
good because spikes in blood glucose levels will double a person's chances of dying from heart attacks and strokes.[8]

Moreover, Professor Christiansen also showed that, over the

FIGURE 1.2A
Plasma glucose levels in type 2 diabetics who eat breakfast.

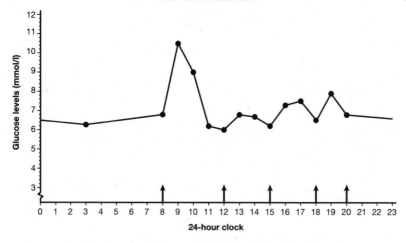

13 patients were studied on four occasions, and their results averaged.
The arrows indicate that breakfast was served at 8.00, lunch at 12.00,
a snack at 15.00, dinner at 18.00 and supper at 20.00.

rest of the day, the breakfast eaters' blood glucose levels remain volatile; and such volatility not only adds a further risk of the two cardiovascular diseases of heart attacks and strokes, it also increases the risk of developing a gamut of diabetic complications including blindness, renal failure and the need for limb amputations.[9]

Now look at Figure 1.2B. On the days the diabetics ate no breakfast, they enjoyed mornings of beautifully falling blood glucose levels. On those days they ate bigger lunches and dinners, so their post-lunch and post-dinner rises were higher than on the days they did eat breakfast, but those rises were gentler and therefore safer than the post-breakfast spikes they had thus avoided. (These subjects also ate two snacks a day, but that doesn't change this analysis.)

Professor Christiansen's data and my own experience with my glucometer are, therefore, comparable, and Professor Christiansen has confirmed my unexpected finding that, for type 2

FIGURE 1.2B
Plasma glucose levels in type 2 diabetics who do not eat breakfast.

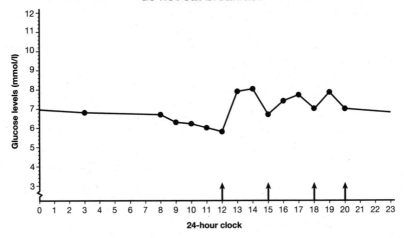

13 patients were studied on four occasions, and their results averaged. Lunch was served at 12.00, a snack at 15.00, dinner at 18.00 and supper at 20.00.

diabetics at least, breakfast is a dangerous meal. As readers of Professor Christiansen's paper will discover, he was equally surprised by the finding, and like me he concluded that type 2 diabetics should skip breakfast.

So, why was I told to eat breakfast?

Box 1: Glucometers and type 2 diabetes

Normally doctors won't give glucometers to patients with type 2 diabetes (only type 1s get them). Here is the recommendation from NICE (the National Institute for Health and Care Excellence) which is the quango that advises doctors on how to treat their patients: 'Do not routinely offer self-monitoring of blood glucose levels for adults with type 2 diabetes.'[10]

NICE gives this advice because of research that suggests that self-monitoring does not benefit type 2 diabetics,[11] but I don't trust that research. Consider slimming and self-weighing. It makes sense that people who weigh themselves regularly would eat less and would lose more weight than people who do not weigh themselves, and although some researchers disagree,[12] most researchers find exactly that.[13] Equally, people who use fitness trackers to monitor their own exercise would be expected to walk more every day, which is what researchers find.[14] Correspondingly, I would expect diabetics who monitor their own blood glucose levels also to improve their control.

As would Diabetes UK, and though it may be unsound on breakfast, it is a superb patients' advocate, and it is shocked that type 2s are not routinely given glucometers. Diabetes UK admits that patients who self-monitor will 'commonly' fail to act on the results of their glucometer readings (thus rendering the blood tests futile), but that failure, it explains, arises only because of patients' 'lack of education in how to interpret them'. That lack of education, moreover, has not been helped by 'a lack of interest in the results from health care professionals'. Consequently, Diabetes UK says, the self-monitoring of blood glucose levels has failed only because 'the professionals expect the patients to self-manage' while the 'patients expect the health care professionals to use the results.'[15]

But I am not only a researcher who has specialised in the biochemistry of glucose and fats, I am also a medical doctor, so I needed no education in interpreting blood glucose levels, and I was grateful for the glucometer my doctor proffered, which allowed me to take control of my diabetes and which also allowed me to discover that the conventional advice was simply wrong. Yet even for non-biochemists and non-doctors the necessary level of education is actually modest, and it should be extended to all patients with type 2 diabetes, so that they too can optimise their diets. It was thanks to his pioneering use of the personal glucometer that the great Dr Bernstein streaked decades ahead of the curve in advocating low-carbohydrate diets for type 1 diabetics,[16] and now we need a Dr Bernstein for type 2s.

Glucometers and their strips can be bought at any pharmacy – no prescriptions are necessary – so if you have type 2, and if you do not have a glucometer, let me urge you to buy your own; and in the meanwhile, for want of anything better, let this book be your education. (The real cost of blood glucose measurements comes, incidentally, not from the purchase of the glucometer but from the test strips. I use roughly sixty strips a month, which costs me about £25 a month, which is cheap at the price.)

———————————

PART TWO

The Dubious Advocates
of Breakfast

We all 'know' that breakfast is the most
important meal of the day and that we should
eat it like kings, lunch like princes and dine
like paupers, but we know these things only
because people have told us so.
Who are these people?

2

The glorification of breakfast

Early one morning, some 3,000 years ago, a Greek army idled while two of its generals argued. As Homer recounts in Book 19 of *The Iliad*, Achilles wanted to attack Troy at dawn, but Odysseus urged him not to send his men 'to fight the Trojans fasting, for the battle will be long and furious, so first get your men to eat bread and wine by the ships'.[1]

Odysseus won the argument, and breakfast was duly served to the troops. Achilles refused his portion but, fortunately, the goddess Athena 'dropped nectar and ambrosia into Achilles, so hunger wouldn't weaken him'. Greek soldiers believed in breakfast, as apparently did everybody in Homeric Greece, and Book 16 of *The Odyssey* opens with 'Back at the hut, Odysseus and the noble swineherd had lit a dawn fire and were making breakfast.'[2]

By the classical era in Greece, around 500 BC (BCE), breakfast seems to have consisted of barley bread or pancakes, sometimes dipped in wine, sometimes complemented by figs or olives. The Romans ate a similar breakfast, around dawn, of bread, cheese, olives, salad, nuts, raisins and perhaps cold meat. The Roman army, though, fed its soldiers a hot breakfast of porridge, similar to polenta, made from roasted spelt wheat or barley that was then pounded and cooked in boiling water.

In their patterns of eating the Greeks and Romans were apparently not unusual, and Heather Anderson opened her 2013 book *Breakfast: A History* with: 'Throughout history, most people partook of a simple breakfast . . . ample written record supports the notion that ancient Romans had a three-meals-a-day (plus afternoon snack) routine similar to that of today's United States and Europe.'[3]

But that routine was not imperishable, and it appears that for a thousand years after the fall of the Roman Empire breakfast was skipped in polite Europe. Thus Charlemagne (748–814) was described as being typical in not eating breakfast,[4] while 700 years later a King of France, Francis I (1494–1547), was still saying that people should 'rise at five, dine at nine, sup at five, and couch at nine',[5] and a generation after that the priest William Harrison was reporting in his 1577 *Description of England* that 'the nobility, gentry and students do ordinarily go to dinner at 11 and to supper at 5,'[6] which was reiterated as late as 1602 by Dr Edmund Hollings, the Renaissance dietician.[7] So, what happened to breakfast after the fall of the Roman Empire?

The Church was one of the things that happened. The clerics disapproved of breakfast as self-indulgent, and, inspired by biblical passages such as Ecclesiastes 10:16, 'Woe to thee, O land, when . . . thy princes eat in the morning,' a writer such as Thomas Aquinas could write in his *Summa Theologica* (1265–74) that breakfast represented *praepropere* or the sin of eating too soon, which was a form of gluttony. Breakfast in medieval Europe was largely, therefore, restricted to children, the elderly, the sick – and to working men: it appears that labourers, needing to fuel their labours, would eat in the morning.

Which was the other thing that happened to breakfast after the fall of the Roman Empire, namely the hierarchy of the feudal system. If working men needed to eat breakfast, then grandees were keen not only to skip it but also to be seen to skip it. Medieval aristocrats, therefore, apparently ate breakfast only when they had to exert themselves, perhaps if travelling or going on pilgrimage, whereupon their spiritual advisers discovered that John 21:12 ('Jesus said to them, "Come and have breakfast,"' English Standard Version) did actually license the practice. So in 1255 Henry III of England ordered 6 tuns of wine (2,112 gallons) for his court's breakfasts while on pilgrimage.[8]

Only with the displacement of feudalism by markets was breakfast revived as a regular meal for the socially respectable, and in his popular article 'How the Tudors Invented Breakfast' Dr Ian Mortimer argued that as the market economy spread, and as people thus worked longer and harder, so those people increasingly demanded three meals a day including breakfast.[9] By 1589, therefore, Thomas Cogan, the Manchester physician and schoolmaster, could write in his *Haven of Health* that it was unhealthy to skip breakfast because to 'suffer hunger long filleth the stomack with ill humors'.[10]

Breakfast in England: Margaret Lane, the author of *Jane Austen and Food*, has chronicled how, for the rich, breakfast then evolved: 'Breakfast in Jane Austen's era [she lived between 1775 and 1817] was very different from the cold meat, coarse bread and ale of earlier ages, or the abundance of eggs, kidneys, bacon and so forth under which Victorian sideboards groaned. Rather it was an elegant light meal of toast and rolls, with tea, coffee or chocolate to drink.'[11]

But Austen's era was still socially divided, and to reinforce their superiority the grander classes ate their breakfasts late: 'The planned excursion from Barton Park to Whitwell in *Sense and Sensibility* begins with the whole party assembling at Barton Park for breakfast at ten . . . Jane frequently wrote letters before breakfast. In London she even went shopping.'[12] Dissolute members of the aristocracy might breakfast even later. Roger Carbury in Anthony Trollope's 1875 novel *The Way We Live Now*, 'would come at twelve as Felix generally breakfasted at that hour'.[13]

The late breakfasts, though, pressed up against dinner, which was then eaten in the middle of the day and which was then – as it had been for a thousand years – the biggest meal of the day, so that meal gradually got pushed back. Eventually, as the prosperous classes increasingly enjoyed an evening social life facilitated by candle and other artificial lights, their dinner moved so late as to become an evening meal, largely displacing supper, which was reduced to a bedtime snack. But the lateness of dinner then created a midday gap, which had to be filled by a new meal, which was sometimes called 'nuncheon' after 'noonshine' (in *Sense and Sensibility* Willoughby takes nuncheon in an inn) but which became corrupted to 'luncheon' (in *Pride and Prejudice* Lydia and Kitty order luncheon in an inn).

Recapitulating its origins in a snack, this new meal was initially only a cold spread, but as Anthony Trollope captured in *The Way We Live Now*, it grew: 'There were two dinner parties every day, one at two o'clock called lunch, and the other at eight.'[14] The confusions around the new meal were reflected in 1847 by a fashionable physician, Dr William Robertson, in his *Treatise on Diet and Regimen*: 'that anomalous meal, luncheon, becomes necessary or desirable if the dinner cannot be taken about five hours after the breakfast. If a man . . . cannot dine before five in the evening, he should eat luncheon.'[15]

The working classes, though, continued to eat their dinner in the middle of the day, and some parts of the north of England and Scotland still describe the midday meal as dinner and the evening meal as tea or high tea. To this day many schools describe the ladies who serve lunch as 'dinner ladies'.

Breakfast in America: Heather Anderson reports that, initially, the Americans and Britons shared a common breakfast culture:

> By the middle of the 18th century, England and America alike were basking in the glow of breakfast's budding golden age; matitudinal feasts of mutton chops, bacon, eggs, corn cakes, and muffins – even pies – were favourites of American Founding fathers Benjamin Franklin and Thomas Jefferson . . . Franklin's only complaint was that his co-workers drank too much beer in the morning . . . In well-to-do English households, most days began with porridge, followed by bacon and eggs . . . Soon the Victorian era witnessed the birth

of Britain's greatest (perhaps only) culinary achievement: the
Full Breakfast.*

But as American meals and waistlines expanded, so a reaction
developed, and during the 1830s the Popular Health Movement
arose to advocate a frugal, near-vegetarian diet. In 1863, to help
meet the demand for a more modest lifestyle, Dr James Caleb
Jackson (1811–95), a New York physician, invented Granula,
which consisted of nuggets of bran-rich Graham flour (a type
of wholemeal flour). The first wholegrain breakfast cereal had
arrived.

In the same year, 1863, and emerging in part from the
same Popular Health Movement, the Seventh-day Adventist
Church was established at Battle Creek, Michigan. The Adven-
tists' theology lies outside the purlieus of this book but its
health message is relevant because it promotes a vegetarian,
alcohol- and caffeine-free lifestyle. In 1866 the Church opened
a sanatorium, also at Battle Creek, where its vegetarian teach-
ings were harnessed to cure as well as to prevent disease. Its
therapies were holistic, employing nutrition, enemas and exercise; and it was at the sanatorium, in 1894, that its most famous
superintendent, Dr John Kellogg (1854–1943), invented cornflakes. Dr Jackson's Granula had not been very convenient
(it needed to be soaked overnight) but cornflakes were very

---

* Sir Kenelm Digby (1603–65) is credited with having been the first to
have published, albeit posthumously, in his 1669 *The Closet of the Emi-
nently Learned Sir Kenelme Digbie Kt Opened*, the assertion that 'Two
Poched Eggs with a few fine dry-fryed collops of pure Bacon, are not
bad for break-fast.' Sir Kenelm was the son of the executed Gunpow-
der Plot conspirator Sir Everard Digby, he was a founder of the Royal
Society, and he was an ancestor of Pamela Harriman, née Digby, who
was to marry Winston Churchill's son Randolph. Digby's genius reveals
how unfair Heather Anderson was to suggest that breakfast might be
Britain's only culinary achievement, because a century earlier Cardinal
Wolsey had created another delicious juxtaposition of two comple-
mentary foods, strawberries and cream.

convenient indeed, and with his brother, Will, John Kellogg created the cereal company we know today.

Some of the beliefs of those Popular Health Movement pioneers are now easy to mock. In his 1877 *Plain Facts for Old and
Young* John Kellogg advocated some robust measures against
masturbation:

> To prevent erection the prepuce or foreskin is drawn forward
> over the glans, and the needle to which the wire is attached
> is passed through from one side to another. After drawing the
> wire through, the ends are twisted together and cut off close.
> It is now impossible for an erection to occur . . . In females the
> author has found the application of pure carbolic acid [phenol]
> to the clitoris an excellent means of allaying the abnormal
> excitement.[16]

And in his 1893 *Ladies' Guide in Health and Disease* John Kellogg indeed recommended clitorectomy for nymphomania. An
early example of FGM in the western world. Yet John's views
on masturbation were not an isolated idiosyncrasy, because
they seemingly linked to his views on breakfast: he apparently
trusted that the low levels of cornflake nutrition would inhibit
early morning masturbation. Meat, he believed, fuelled lust:
'Flesh, condiments, eggs, tea, chocolate and all stimulants have
a powerful influence directly on the reproductive organs. They
increase the local supply of blood; and through nervous sym-
pathy with the brain, the passions are aroused.'[17] But cornflakes
would leave a person energetically deprived.[18]

Although he never explicitly marketed cornflakes as an
energy-depleting anti-masturbatory tool, John Kellogg nonetheless conceived breakfast cereals – which are now sold as
nutritionally valuable – to be nutritionally poor. The history of
breakfast is littered with these ironies because, until recently,
opinions emerged out of beliefs, not out of empirical evidence.

John was an intellectual who took ideas seriously. His views
on masturbation were then orthodox, as were his views on
eugenics (he was in favour) and constipation (he was against),

but his brother, Will, was not an intellectual and – to promote their palatability – he put sugar into cornflakes, which John opposed. John lost that fight but it was sincerely fought.

One of their contemporaries, Dr Dewey of Meadville, Pennsylvania, went even further, and in his 1900 book *The No-Breakfast Plan and the Fasting Cure* he advocated skipping breakfast altogether: Dewey wrote that patients who skipped breakfast seemed to make better and faster cures from illnesses than did breakfast eaters.

The revival of breakfast: By the 1920s Dr Dewey seemed to be winning the argument: breakfast in America was apparently declining into little more than a snack. This was a concern to the Beech-Nut Packing Company, which was raising lots of pigs but which was finding too few buyers for its bacon, and it therefore commissioned Edward Bernays to rescue its market.

Bernays, one of the fathers of PR, was the nephew of Sigmund Freud, whose techniques he exploited on behalf of powerful clients, which included American Tobacco (for whom he helped break the taboo against women smoking in public) and the United Fruit Company (for whom he helped engineer the coup that removed the democratically elected president of Guatemala, Jacobo Arbenz Guzman). Bernays, famously, influenced Goebbels, which is no surprise since in his 1928 book *Propaganda* he'd written:

> The conscious and intelligent manipulation of the organised habits and opinions of the masses is an important element in democratic society. Those who manipulate this unseen mechanism of society constitute an invisible government which is the true ruling power of our country . . . We are governed, our minds are molded, our tastes formed, our ideas suggested, largely by men we have never heard of.[19]

One opinion of the masses that Bernays resolved to manipulate was their commitment to a 'very light breakfast of coffee, with maybe a roll and orange juice', which he sought to replace 'with a heavy breakfast'; and in a film (still available as a video on the web)[20] Bernays explained how he mobilised 4,500 doctors to publicly support Beech-Nut's faith in heavy breakfasts.* In the words of Dr Kaori O'Connor, a social anthropologist at University College London and the author of the 2013 book *The English Breakfast: The Biography of an English Meal*: 'the idea that [breakfast] is healthy in its own right was laid on a plate for us by marketing companies. And, by and large, we've gobbled it up.'[21]

The breakfast mantras: It was in 1847, in the fourth edition of his *Treatise on Diet and Regimen*, that Dr William Robertson, who practised medicine in Buxton, Derbyshire, UK, wrote that 'Breakfast should always be an important, if not the most important, meal of the day.'[22] As I have already noted, Dr Robertson was a prominent physician, so it behoves us to ask: what research led him to coin that momentous phrase? Which careful observations, which controlled experiments, underpinned that weighty idiom? Well, this is what he wrote: 'Breakfast is very properly made to consist of a considerable proportion of liquids, to supply the loss of the fluids of the body during the hours of sleep.'

Eh? It is true we lose water through our lungs and sweat glands as we sleep, but why was Dr Robertson so fixated on that? Well, Dr Robertson was a *water* physician: he practised

---

* If you're surprised that so many doctors would support such an assertion, think on this: a 2015 survey by Credit Suisse found that 54 per cent of doctors believe that eating cholesterol-rich food not only raises blood levels of cholesterol but also damages the heart, even though these statements were discredited forty years ago (see later) and were disowned even by their original progenitor, Ancel Keys. In the words of the survey: 'This is a clear example of the level of misinformation that exists among doctors' (Credit Suisse Research Institute (September 2015), 'Fat: The New Health Paradigm', http://publications. credit-suisse.com/tasks/render/file/index.cfm? fileid=9163B920-CAEF-91FB-EE5769786A03D76E. Accessed April 2016).

in Buxton, which was a spa town whose waters were believed to cure myriad diseases, so of course Dr Robertson believed that water lay at the heart of health and illness. But that belief – which is barely more advanced than Hippocrates' belief in the four humours – is an absurdity. Yet Dr Robertson was no one-trick pony, and he also believed that 'the nervous system is restored by sleep to its fullest power and activity,' and that we should therefore eat early 'before the nervous system has become expended by its mental and physical labours', which is a further absurdity.

The other great breakfast mantra is, of course, Adelle Davis's injunction to 'Eat breakfast like a king, lunch like a prince, and dinner like a pauper.'[23] Adelle Davis (1904–74) was the most popular nutritionist in America of her day, and though she was a controversial figure who was regularly accused of misusing science to promote dietary fads, she sold over 10 million copies of books with titles such as *Let's Eat Right to Keep Fit* (1954). As to her famous mantra, let us ask: what was the thinking behind it? Did it emerge from the systematic scientific study of a problem that is still urgent today, or did it emerge out of a health scare that has since been discredited?

Post-war, America went through a strange panic over low blood sugar levels, and a charity called the Hypoglycemia Foundation claimed that 'There is probably no illness today which causes so much widespread suffering, so much inefficiency and loss of time, so many accidents, so many family breakups and so many suicides as hypoglycemia.'[24]

The media followed suit, and a magazine such as *Family Circle* could in June 1965 assert that 'millions among us . . . suffer unknowingly from low blood sugar' while *Town and Country* could state in June 1971 that 'ten million Americans have hypoglycaemia.' Respected professionals fed the national anxiety, and a psychiatrist wrote that

'about half of the people I see for psychiatric problems have abnormal blood sugar . . . the incidence in schizophrenia is high and in neuroses even higher.'[25]

Adelle Davis herself asserted that 'irritability resulting from low blood sugar can be a factor in divorces.'[26]

It is rare for a bizarre new idea to emerge without some-one, somewhere, profiting from it, and it appears that the hypoglycaemia scare coincided with the discovery that adre-nal extracts – which were expensive and therefore profitable to administer – could 'cure' hypoglycaemia; but the respect-able authorities rallied against the charlatans, and in 1973 the American Medical Association, the American Diabetes Asso-ciation and the Endocrine Society published a joint statement saying that few Americans suffer from low blood sugar levels, which in any case were not dangerous:

Statement on Hypoglycemia

Recent publicity in the popular press has led the public to believe that the occurrence of hypoglycemia is high in this country and that many of the symptoms that affect the American population are not recognised as being caused by this condition. These claims are not supported by the medical evidence.[27]

Adelle Davis, therefore, coined her great aphorism to address a non-problem: she knew that the blood sugar levels of break-fast skippers fell gently during the mornings,[28] and since raised blood sugar levels are one of the great killers of our time, so the same data that inspired Davis's mantra should now inspire its revision: *Eat breakfast like a pauper.*

We see, therefore, that the two popular breakfast mantras were coined to address the non-problems of night-time dehy-dration, night-time starvation, brain fatigue and rampant hypoglycaemia, yet those mantras remain so potent that many people today believe they have a metabolic duty to eat break-fast. In a world where millions of people overeat, their pushing themselves to eat a meal they might otherwise skip is not a trivial matter.

The Mediterranean breakfast: Judging by the longevities of the people who eat it, the Mediterranean diet is healthier than that of northern Europe or North America, and in his 2003 book *Food in Early Modern Europe* Ken Alabala, professor of history at the University of the Pacific, California, notes that in southern Europe breakfast never really developed: 'In countries where the evening meal was larger, breakfast did not become important. In southern Europe it is still not a proper meal, but merely coffee and perhaps a piece of bread or pastry. In England and the north [of Europe] the pattern was quite different.'[29]

As a group of senior Italian nutritionists wrote in 2009: 'Every morning, most [Italian] adults just drink a cup of coffee or a cappuccino.'[30]

Yet as the World Health Organization, the United Nations and the CIA have all confirmed, the Italians live longer than either the British or the Americans.[31] That doesn't, of course, prove that breakfast is bad for you, but it does weaken the suggestion that good health is impossible without it.

Overview: When, in Tudor times, the European aristocracy ceased to skip breakfast, certain wise contemporaries expressed alarm. In 1542 the celebrated physician Andrew Boorde wrote in his *Dietary of Health* that 'A labourer may eat three times a day but two meals a day are adequate for a rest man.'[32]

Why? Because, Boorde said, 'repletion shortens a man's life.'[33] Equally, in his *Naturall and Artificial Directions for Health* of 1602,[34] the scholar William Vaughan advised us to:

'eat three meals a day until you come to the age of 40 years,'[35]

which was echoed by Sir John Harington (1560–1612):

'feed only twice a day when you are at man's age.'[36]

As we'll discover, breakfast is dangerous because it is eaten when the body is most insulin-resistant, and, as we'll also discover, the people who are most at risk of insulin-resistance are those who are over 45 years old and physically inactive. We might do worse than recapitulate the sixteenth-century wisdom of Dr Boorde and others.

Our best guide to breakfast may be Franz Kafka, who in his 1915 book *Metamorphosis* described how 'for Gregor's father, breakfast was the most important meal of the day.'[37] This description is often invoked by pro-breakfast scientists,[38] but their confidence is misplaced because the full quote is: 'The washing up from breakfast lay on the table; there was so much of it because, for Gregor's father, breakfast was the most important meal of the day, and he would stretch it out for several hours as he sat reading a number of different newspapers.' Kafka is actually telling us that Gregor's father is a jerk, who won't work to support his family but who will nonetheless lash out at Gregor, the family breadwinner.

And with that image of breakfast as the meal of moral degenerates, I shall end this review of its history.

3

Breakfast in an age of commercial science

An article published in 1917 in *Good Health*, the self-proclaimed 'oldest health magazine in the world', reiterated that 'breakfast is the most important meal of the day,'[1] and *Good Health* was edited by Dr John Kellogg. So here's the worry. Type the popular mantras into Google today, and you discover that many of the studies asserting them are supported and funded by the manufacturers of breakfast cereals.

As a simple experiment, on 24 October 2015 I typed 'breakfast' into Google Scholar and downloaded the first ten papers that were medical or biological and which were fully accessible online. Of those ten papers, would you like to guess how many were funded, at least in part, by Kellogg, General Mills, Nestlé or some other food company? The answer is given in the footnote.*

---

* The ten papers were (1) G.C. Rampersaud et al. (2005), *J Am Diet Assoc* 105: 743–60, (2) M.R. Malinow et al. (1998), *N Engl J Med* 338: 1009–15, (3) A.M. Siega-Riz et al. (1998), *Am J Clin Nutr* 67 (suppl): 748S–56S, (4) A. Keski-Rahkonen et al. (2003), *Eur J Clin Nutr* 57: 842–53, (5) H.R. Wyatt et al. (2002), *Obes Res* 10: 78–82, (6) C.S. Berkey et al. (2003), *Int J Obes* 27: 1258–66, (7) R.E. Kleinman et al. (2002), *Ann Nutr Metab* 46 (suppl 1): 24–30, (8) E. Pollitt, R. Mathews (1998), *Am J Clin Nutr* 67 (suppl): 804S–13S, (9) D. Benton, P.Y. Parker (1998), *Am J Clin Nutr* 67 (suppl): 772S–8S, (10) D.T. Simeon, S. Grantham-McGregor (1989), *Am J Clin Nutr* 49: 646–53.

Breakfast is big business: global breakfast cereal sales are expected to reach $43.2 billion annually by 2019, up from $32.5 billion in 2012, and the North American market alone was worth $13.9 billion in 2012. But that North American market is now mature, which is why manufacturers now target the emerging world.[2] Of course they do: the breakfast cereal business is a great business; the raw product (grain or rice) is cheap but the final product on the supermarket shelves is not so cheap.

The fast food breakfast market is also big and growing. Dominated by McDonald's, it was worth $31.7 billion in 2012 in North America, and between 2007 and 2012 its sales increased by 4.8 per cent annually.[3] Fast food = meat = protein, and that message is now so strong that Kellogg's has entered that market, to sell Kellogg's Special K Flatbread Breakfast Sandwich Sausage, Egg and Cheese.[4] These sandwiches, which are designed to be microwaved at home, look to English eyes like hamburgers. They are so small as to each deliver only 240 calories, but each sandwich also delivers 820 mg sodium (over 2 g of actual salt) which is a third of the daily recommended intake, and as most people would eat two Flatbread Sandwiches for breakfast, they will not only have consumed a gratuitous meal, they will also have consumed two-thirds of their daily allowance for salt before leaving the house in the morning.[5] Still, the packet boasts a pretty photograph of two slices of orange placed alongside the Kellogg's Special K Flatbread Breakfast Sandwich Sausage, Egg and Cheese.

Research funded by companies tends to produce results that

All ten papers were supportive of breakfast, and of the eight papers that disclosed their funding sources (two didn't, which is odd), seven received at least some funding from industry. The sources of funding included Kellogg, General Mills, Nestlé and Friehofer's Baking Company via Project Bread/the Walk for Hunger.

This survey of the top ten Google Scholar papers is obviously simplistic, but nonetheless it does give an indication not only of the academic consensus in favour of breakfast but also of the degree of the industrial support for breakfast scholarship and research.

are favourable to those companies: there will rarely be actual dishonesty on the part of the scientists, but nonetheless a bias can creep into the published findings. Consider the pharmaceutical industry. There is a class of drugs known as 'calcium-channel antagonists' that are prescribed for heart disease, and over the years at least seventy clinical studies on these drugs have been published by university professors and practising doctors. Some of those studies were funded by the manufacturers, while others were funded by independent sources including charities, government research agencies and hospitals, and in 1998 a group of investigators from the University of Toronto found: 'A strong association between scientists' opinions about safety and their financial relationships with the manufacturers. Supportive scientists were much more likely than critical scientists to have financial associations with the manufacturers.'[6]

University professors and practising doctors, therefore, publish findings that support their sources of research money. Repeated surveys of scientists' publications have confirmed this finding, which is why journals now require the authors of papers to list their sources of research income and consultancies. Yet such listings can still leave the reader adrift: does an industrial association negate a researcher's work, or can they be trusted anyway?

The food and drinks companies will also manipulate publication. David Ludwig is a hero in the battle against obesity. He is a professor of paediatrics at Harvard and an author of the 2007 book *Ending the Food Fight: Guide Your Child to a Healthy Weight in a Fast Food/Fake Food World*. He is also an author of a study that found that research papers that have been funded, at least in part, by the drinks manufacturers are four to eight times more likely to report good news about commercial drinks than those that were funded independently. No research paper, moreover, that was funded wholly by the drinks manufacturers reported any bad news.* Since so many papers

---

* Pharmaceutical companies, too, will try not to publish inconvenient results, and a recent survey showed how, five years after they had been

on drinks are funded by the manufacturers, Ludwig concluded that the whole field of study has been biased.[7]

So we have to be careful: breakfast studies have been infused by industrially funded science, and we may be at the same stage in their development as cigarette studies were before 1950, when Richard Doll and Bradford Hill discovered the link between smoking and lung cancer. Before 1950, and even for a time afterwards, that field was dominated by academic papers, sponsored by the tobacco companies, that proclaimed the health benefits of cigarettes and which then supported the subsequent advertising ('More doctors smoke Camels than any other cigarette', 'L&M Filters are just what the doctor ordered', 'Reach for a Lucky instead of a sweet').

Industrial money gets into surprising places. Even the great charities accept commercial funding: so Diabetes UK charges companies between £10,000 and £25,000 p.a. for using the Diabetes UK logo and name, while in 2013 at least twelve companies gave the American Diabetes Association more than $500,000. The charities do invaluable work, so they need support, and though it is perhaps a shame they solicit money from industry, they are nonetheless sensible of the risks and they implement scrupulous ethical policies. Which can be very effective. In 2013, for example, Dr Heather Leidy and her colleagues from the University of Missouri published a paper with a convoluted title: 'Beneficial effects of a higher-protein breakfast on the appetitive, hormonal, and neural signals controlling energy intake regulation in overweight/obese, "breakfast skipping," late-adolescent girls'.[8]

And though Dr Leidy acknowledged that her study was supported by the beef and egg producer associations, she also wrote

---

completed, 23 per cent of clinical trials had not been published (V.S. Moorthy et al. (2015), 'Rationale for WHO's new position calling for prompt reporting and public disclosure of interventional clinical trial results', *PLOS Med* 12: e1001819). For a comprehensive survey see Ben Goldacre's 2013 book *Bad Pharma: How Medicine is Broken, and How We Can Fix It*, Fourth Estate, London.

PART THREE

Breakfast Myths

There are so many breakfast myths that
I hardly know which ones to demolish first,
but here we go.

(Please note: we're not looking at the
diabetic breakfast here, we're looking at
everybody's breakfast. The diabetic breakfast
may have got me involved, but breakfast
is bigger than diabetes.)

4

Myth No. 1: Breakfast cereals are healthy

Oh no they're not. They're largely carbohydrates befouled by sugar, and it is hard to think of a worse morning meal. In 2006 the British consumer protection magazine *Which?* examined 275 different breakfast cereals, finding that 'Nearly 90 per cent of the cereals in our sample that targeted children were high in sugar, 13 per cent were high in salt and 10 per cent were high in saturated fat.' The report was entitled *Cereal Re-offenders*, referring to the reluctance of the manufacturers to respond to repeated criticisms.[1]

And though the manufacturers may add nutrients to their products, they will first have removed them: here is Felicity Lawrence's account in her 2008 book *Eat Your Heart Out* of the denuding of cornflake nourishment:

> Cornflakes are generally made by breaking corn kernels into smaller grits which are then steam cooked in batches of up to a tonne under pressure of about 20lbs per square inch. The nutritious germ with its essential fats is first removed because, as the Kellogg brothers discovered all that time ago, it goes rancid over time and gets in the way of long shelf life. Flavourings, vitamins to replace those lost in processing and sugar may be added at this stage.[2]

Consider niacin (vitamin B3). A deficiency of niacin causes a disease called pellagra, which is an unpleasant condition known for the four Ds: diarrhoea, dermatitis, dementia and death. Pellagra was once epidemic in the American south, and between 1905 and 1940 some 3 million people developed it, of whom about 100,000 died.[3] Because niacin is found in meat, fish, eggs, fruit, vegetables, nuts, whole grains, fungi, beer and yeast extracts such as Marmite, pellagra is a disease of a very deficient diet, and the epidemic of the American south developed only because many of the inhabitants were so poor that they subsisted on a diet primarily of maize (corn) that had been 'de-germed' during its preparation. The de-germination removed the niacin from the cornmeal.*

Partly because the folk memory of the pellagra epidemic has not been lost, and partly because niacin is cheap, the manufacturers of breakfast cereal now boast of how much of it they add, voluntarily, to their products. But, actually, too much is added, and if children today consumed no niacin-fortified foods, only 2.9 per cent of them would consume less than the EAR (Estimated Average Requirement). But currently 28 per cent of American children aged 2 to 8 years old ingest more than the recommended UL (upper limit) – and 2.9 per cent of children consuming less than the EAR may represent less of a public health risk than 28 per cent of them consuming more than the UL.[4]

Other cereal supplements, too, have caused concern. Some manufacturers fortify their products with iron, and in consequence some children consume toxic amounts of it. And in consequence of that, certain countries such as Norway now

---

* By 1890, the USA had the highest GDP per capita in the world (A. Maddison (1982), *Phases of Capitalist Development*, Oxford University Press) so the poverty of the deep south leading to the pellagra epidemic surely needs explaining. In his 1999 book *Development as Freedom* (Oxford University Press, Oxford and New York) the Nobel laureate Amartya Sen wrote that 'No famine has ever taken place in the history of the world in a functioning democracy,' so presumably the pellagra epidemic reflected the workings of the Jim Crow laws in pre-empting the development of a fully functioning democracy in the Dixie states.

ban the fortification of breakfast cereals with iron. The authors of a recent study concluded that: 'Obtaining recommended daily allowances (RDAs) and adequate intakes (AIs) from non-fortified food continues to have the advantage of (i) providing intakes of other potential nutrients and food components, and (ii) potentially enhancing intakes through simultaneous interactions with other nutrients.'[5] Which in English says: 'Eat natural, not artificial, food. Avoid breakfast cereals.'

If breakfast cereals were replaced by unprocessed, more natural foods, children would be healthier: after all, the consumption of ready-to-eat cereals is predominantly an English-speaking phenomenon, and there is no systematic evidence that non-Anglophonic children suffer for not consuming them.

The unhealthiness of breakfast cereals has long inspired humour, and in his 1975 novel *Changing Places* David Lodge wrote that the campus newspaper: 'had recently reported an experiment in which rats fed on cornflake packets had proved healthier than rats fed on the cornflakes'.[6]

And this humour is translating into consumer resistance: Euromonitor International, the marketing company, report that since 2012 breakfast cereal sales in countries such as the USA and UK have fallen by at least 1 per cent a year; and the decline is predicted to continue as consumers increasingly switch to yoghurt, fresh fruits and other protein-based, more natural, low-carbohydrate, low-sugar products.[7]

The US Department of Agriculture continues to defend breakfast cereals as becoming ever healthier,[8] but consumers are, rightly, resisting the corporate message.

Breakfast cereals and Caucasians

Breakfast cereals are a largely Anglophonic phenomenon in part because they are generally served with milk, and milk is a challenge to most non-Caucasian adults: whereas 90 per cent of northern Europeans can drink half a pint of milk without feeling sick, only

40 per cent of southern Europeans and only 35 per cent of the rest of the world can do so. Milk was intended by nature, of course, to be drunk only by infants, and it contains a sugar, lactose, that can normally be absorbed with comfort only by infants because only infant guts express an enzyme, lactase, by which to digest it. Most humans lose the lactase enzyme on leaving infancy but, around 6,500 years ago, Caucasians acquired a mutation by which adults retain it. Caucasians retain the lactase enzyme because, by helping them consume animal milk, which is rich in vitamin D, it helped pre-empt the rickets that bedevilled life in the sun-deprived north of Europe.[9] It was at the same time, some 6,500 or so years ago, that Caucasians also acquired the mutations by which their skin turned white, the better to convert sunshine into vitamin D.

Although lactase mutations have developed independently in certain other ethnic groups, particularly in those that herd sheep, goats and cattle, the adults of most ethnic groups (the Chinese, for example) remain milk-intolerant. Cheese and yoghurt, incidentally, are the products of bacterial fermentation, which breaks down much of the lactose, which is why those foods can be eaten by adults of all ethnic groups.[10]

Globally, there is a good correlation between national rates of milk consumption and height: thus the Dutch and Scandinavians drink the most milk per capita[11] and they are among the tallest people in the world (the average Dutch man now stands at 6 feet 1 inch, 1.84 metres; average Dutch woman 5 feet 7 inches, 1.71 metres). Milk seems to be good for you: it's the cereals they dunk that do the damage.

5

Myth No. 2:
Breakfast is good for the brain

Really? It is widely supposed that children and adolescents must do better at school, cognition-wise, if they eat breakfast, yet the conclusions of the most systematic reviews of the field are surprisingly tentative. So two comprehensive reviews of forty-five studies conducted between 1950 and 2008 concluded that eating breakfast seems to benefit the education only of children from deprived homes – and not necessarily because their brains need the morning calories but perhaps because children from deprived homes, on being lured to school by free food programmes, cannot then truant.[1]

If the evidence for breakfast benefiting the cognition of children is weak, it is even weaker for adults. In 1992 a study from the Department of Psychology, Cardiff University, Wales, found that, though breakfast seemed to improve adults' morning 'recognition memory' and 'logical reasoning', it impaired their afternoon 'semantic processing'.[2] In 1994 the Cardiff psychologists found that breakfast improved 'free recall' and 'recognition memory', had no effect on 'semantic memory', but impaired 'logical reasoning'.[3]

So eating breakfast seems to improve some aspects of brain function yet impair others, and the general lack of certainty over what – if anything – breakfast does systematically to brain function was revealed by a 2014 review of the fifteen most careful research papers in children and adults which concluded that: 'There is insufficient quantity and consistency among studies to draw firm conclusions.'[4]

But researchers need not be restricted to merely observing populations, they can also do experiments, and in 2014 a group from Utrecht, in the Netherlands, published a paper with the exciting title of 'Always gamble on an empty stomach: hunger is associated with advantageous decision making'.[5] Using the Iowa Gambling Task as a model for 'complex decision tasks with uncertain outcomes', the Utrecht team found that, when thirty university students skipped breakfast, they performed better in standard psychological tests that modelled decision-making and risk-taking. Leaders, the paper concluded, should skip breakfast.

Free school breakfasts

The first free school breakfasts were served by the School Funds Societies in Paris in 1867, and by 1890 a free breakfast programme in Birmingham, England, was providing children with 'a substantial hunk of bread and a cup of warm milk' before the first class. By the 1920s Norwegian schoolchildren were enjoying the Oslo Breakfast of rye biscuit, brown bread, butter or margarine fortified with vitamins, whey cheese, cod liver oil paste, a generous bottle of milk, raw carrot, an apple and half an orange, and by the twenties such government largesse was becoming typical throughout Europe.

The USA, though, remained committed to laissez-faire, private philanthropy and states' rights, and these seem to have worked well: 'as early as 1905 charitable religious foundations began offering free breakfasts in churches to needy schoolchildren.'[6] The inspirer of these initiatives was the journalist Albert Shaw, who in 1891 claimed with no evidence that 'to drive children into school to fill their heads when they have nothing in their stomachs is like pouring water into a sieve.'[7] The federal government eventually sought permanent congressional authorisation for its School Breakfast Program only as late as 1975, not because the contemporary providers had failed but, rather, because their actions – and one initiative in particular – had proved too successful.

By 1970, though it had been launched only two years earlier, the Black Panther Party's 'Free Children's Breakfast Program' was feeding thousands of African-American children in church kitchens. It was also using those breakfasts to teach the Panthers' view of black history. As Huey Newton and Nik Heynen have argued, it was not its militancy but, rather, the success of its breakfast-time educational programmes that led J. Edgar Hoover to declare that 'the Black Panther Party, without question, represents the greatest threat to the internal security of the country.'[8] To crowd out the party's educational programmes, the federal government understood it first had to crowd out its free eggs, bacon, grits, toast and orange juice.

6

Myth No. 3: Breakfast is slimming

Pundit after pundit asserts that breakfast produces satiety (from the Latin *satis*, enough). Breakfast, it is claimed, fills people's stomachs and raises their blood sugar levels so they eat less at subsequent meals. Is this true?

There are of course peer-reviewed scientific papers that make such assertions, and a man who has written many of them is Dr John de Castro, a Texas psychologist, who in 2004 wrote: 'we found that when individual subjects ate a larger than mean proportion of their total intake in the morning, they ate significantly less over the entire day.'[1] Which *apparently* means that the more someone eats at breakfast, the less they eat during the rest of the day. De Castro attributed this to satiety. Here is his model:

Eat breakfast → satiety → eat less at lunch → lose weight

This is a powerful model, which at first sight seems to make sense. But most scientists find the exact opposite. In a recent study David Levitsky and Carly Pacanowski of Cornell University, New York, showed that when subjects were provided with light breakfasts (approx. 350 calories) their intake at lunch was completely unchanged: i.e. those 350 breakfast calories did not cause a compensatory fall in lunch calories, so on eating breakfast their daily intake went up by 350 calories. Moreover, when the subjects ate full breakfasts of around 624 calories, they reduced their lunch calories by only about 144 calories, causing a net increase of 480 calories a day.[2] No wonder Levitsky and Pacanowski concluded that 'skipping breakfast may be an effective means to reduce energy intake.' The Levitsky and Pacanowski model is, therefore:

Skip breakfast → consume less food → reduce energy intake

or vice versa

Eat breakfast → consume more food → increase energy intake

And what made Levitsky and Pacanowski's study so significant is that they showed that 'these data are consistent with published literature.' That is to say there is widespread agreement that de Castro's satiety hypothesis is wrong and that eating breakfast increases energy intake.

Indeed, an overview of forty-seven of the most authoritative breakfast studies performed between 1952 and 2003 confirmed that around 20 per cent of children and adults skip breakfast, and that 'breakfast eaters generally consumed more daily calories.'[3] So, contrary to myth, eating breakfast piles on the calories. How then do we account for de Castro's finding that 'when individual subjects ate a larger than mean proportion of their total intake in the morning, they ate significantly less over the entire day'?

Dramatically, Dr Volker Schusdziarra and his colleagues from the obesity clinic at the Technical University of Munich in Germany dismiss de Castro's breakfast conclusions as a statistical illusion.[4] On studying a cohort of subjects, Dr Schusdziarra found that, left to their own devices, people tend to eat fairly consistently in the mornings (i.e. breakfast is a relatively fixed-sized meal, because it is a habit) but people tend to eat *in*consistently later in the day: on some days (for whatever reason – Aunt Flo's birthday party, a celebratory restaurant meal) people will eat more at lunch and dinner, whereas on other days (for whatever reason – not feeling well, being rushed at work) people will eat less at lunch and dinner.

Yet because the intake at breakfast is reasonably fixed, on the days that people ate large lunches and dinners, the *proportion* of their food intake from breakfast was small, while on the days they ate small lunches and dinners, the *proportion* of their food intake from breakfast was large. So it *looks* as if:

small breakfasts ➜ large overall food intake

And

large breakfasts ➜ small overall food intake

But these are illusions based on the greater variability of consumption at lunch and dinner, and the real model is:

large intake at lunch   ➜   breakfasts correspondingly
and dinner   small, relatively

And

small intake at lunch   ➜   breakfasts correspondingly
and dinner   large, relatively

Schusdziarra was rightly respectful of de Castro's data; it was only his interpretation he challenged. And this, as will be seen, is the theme of this book: the accumulated breakfast data of literally hundreds of scientists is almost always sound (it's amazing how much breakfast research has been performed), but the findings have been systematically misinterpreted.

Satiety and social eating

Satiety can of course be real. Children up to the age of 3 will eat only in response to satiety signals, but by the age of 5 their appetites are already being modified by other signals – social signals. So Brian Wansink of the Cornell University Food and Brand Laboratory reported in his 2006 book *Mindless Eating* that when researchers from Pennsylvania State University:

> gave three- or five-year-old children either medium-size or large-size servings of macaroni and cheese, the three-year-olds ate the same amount regardless of what they were given. They ate until they were full and then they stopped. [But] the five-year-olds rose to the occasion and ate 26 percent more when they were given bigger servings. Almost exactly the same thing happens to adults. We let the size of the serving influence how much we eat.[5]

In her 2011 book *Eat What You Love, Love What You Eat* Dr Michelle May listed the social and psychological signals that can override satiety in encouraging us to overeat.[6] These include loneliness, depression, anxiety, stress and boredom. Or, in the words of Comic Book Guy from the 1997 episode of *The Simpsons* (#8.17), 'My Sister, My Sitter': 'Loneliness and cheeseburgers are a dangerous mix.'

Distraction, too, can be a major eating stimulant: a recent overview of twenty-four separate research papers concluded that people who eat while being distracted (munching crisps while watching television, say) increase their food intake on average by 76 per cent.[7] This is because distracted eaters not only eat mindlessly but also retain little memory of having eaten, so they approach their next meal assuming they must be hungry. There is wisdom behind the old injunction of 'not eating between meals'.

Another social signal is company: in a series of studies for which he is rightly well known, John de Castro reported that, if you eat with one other person, your consumption goes up by 35 per cent; if you eat with three other people, your consumption goes up by 75 per cent; and if you eat with six other people your consumption goes up by 96 per cent.[8] Which is why Wansink wrote in *Mindless Eating* that weight 'can be contagious'.[9]

And we humans are not the only social animal whose eating is stimulated by company: as long ago as 1929 it was discovered that, when a solitary chicken was replete and had stopped eating, the admission of another chicken into its cage would prompt it to start eating again.[10] The same behaviour is true of pigs, fish, rats, gerbils, puppies and primates. Social animals eat socially. Brian Wansink has even shown that the amount of food we order in a restaurant is influenced by the mass of the waiter: 'diners were . . . four times more likely to order desserts . . . when served by heavy wait staff with high body mass indices.'[11]

Our species has been honed by aeons of evolution to seek social approval, so our eating is determined as much by our social and psychological choices as by our satiety, which we can override in daily practice.

(In this book I follow academic fashion in describing the extraordinary contemporary incidence of obesity and diabetes as 'epidemic' or 'pandemic'. Originally, epidemics and pandemics were defined as diseases that spread from person to person, yet because overeating is socially transmittable, the use of the terms to describe obesity and diabetes may be defensible.)

An exception: Although humans generally eat more in company, a Vanderbilt University research group showed in a 'get-acquainted' session in a psychology laboratory that human females – unlike human males – will snack up to 75 per cent less in the presence of a desirable member of the opposite sex, which caused the researchers to speculate on the role of feminine self-presentation in the development of anorexia.[12] This female trait was satirised by Aldous Huxley in chapter 19 of his 1921 novel *Crome Yellow*:

> He noticed with surprise and a certain solicitous distress that Miss Emmeline's appetite was poor, that it didn't, in fact, exist. Two spoonfuls of soup, a morsel of fish, no bird, no meat, three grapes – that was her whole dinner . . .
>
> 'Pray, don't talk to me of eating,' said Emmeline, drooping like a sensitive plant. 'We find it so coarse, so unspiritual, my sisters and I.'

But some time later the protagonist finds a secret door, which he opens to find the sisters tucking into a good lunch. The protagonist promptly blackmails one of the sisters, Georgiana, into marrying him.

———————————

PART FOUR

The Breakfast Paradox

Breakfast eaters are slimmer than breakfast skippers: does this mean we should eat breakfast? (Hint: no.)

7

Yo-yo dieting

Studies on populations generally find that people who eat breakfast are thinner than people who skip it.[1] Yet those self-same studies generally also find that people who eat breakfast consume more calories over the course of the day than do skippers. How can we reconcile these data?

Well, one of the reasons people skip breakfast is that they're dieters. And who diets? Large people. So an Australian survey of 699 13-year-olds, 12 per cent of whom skipped breakfast, found that girls who believe themselves to be fat will go on weight-loss diets, and they will do so in part by skipping breakfast.[2]

The girls in that Australian study may, of course, have had false body images, and they may not have been large, but a study on female college students in North Carolina found that 48 per cent of the obese ones had skipped breakfast, as opposed to only 40 per cent of the overweight ones and just 27 per cent of the normally weighted ones.[3] So large people do indeed skip breakfast.

That particular North Carolina study covered only 166 subjects, so it missed being statistically significant ($p<0.09$ in the jargon), but multiple surveys have confirmed that skipping breakfast is a common reaction to overweight and obesity.[4] Consequently, large people will diet and will lose weight but – and here comes a key point – dieters generally fail to keep down their weight, and in so-called yo-yo dieting they tend to revert to being large.[5] So as people cycle between:

- being large and so losing weight by skipping breakfast
- being slim and so eating breakfast again

we have found one resolution to the breakfast/body weight paradox. I.e. when people are large they skip breakfast and eat less (so largeness is associated with skipping breakfast) but when people have slimmed down they eat breakfast and other meals again and, unfortunately, put the weight back on (so slimness is associated with eating breakfast). But it's not the eating of breakfast that determines weight, it's weight that determines the eating of breakfast. I.e., it's not:

eat breakfast → consume more → paradoxically
                 calories   be slim
or
skip breakfast → consume fewer → paradoxically
                 calories   be large

rather it's:

be slim → can afford to eat breakfast
or
be large → respond by skipping breakfast

Why do dieters return to their previous weight?

Just as Mark Twain is reported to have said that quitting smoking was easy, he'd done it a thousand times, so dieters find it equally easy to lose weight, they've done it a thousand times. But then they put it back on again, and repeated studies have confirmed that 80–90 per cent of dieters revert to their previous weight.[6] At least five reasons have been proffered for this yo-yo dieting: namely (i) pleasure, (ii) the replacement of muscle by fat, (iii) resetting the basal metabolic and exercise rates, (iv) hormones and (v) genes.

Pleasure: Conventional dieting is rarely fun, and the temptation to start eating again at the end of a weight-loss diet is strong, so people who skipped breakfast when dieting will, on breaking their diet, eat it again (thus, incidentally, creating the paradox of large people skipping breakfast and slim ones eating it).

The replacement of muscle by fat: Dieters do not lose only fat: many researchers report that dieters, on losing weight, lose muscle mass as well. But on recovering their weight, former dieters put back more fat than muscle. And because fat consumes less energy than muscle, the former dieter – if they want to maintain a fixed weight – needs to eat less food than before, which they will generally fail to do.

The first study to report this so-called 'preferential restocking of fat tissue on refeeding' was the famous Minnesota starvation study that the now notorious (see later) Ancel Keys performed over 1944/45. Concerned by the mass starvations of the Second World War, and believing (rightly) that they needed to be better understood, Keys recruited thirty-six conscientious objectors (male, lean, aged 22–33) with his celebrated advert, 'Will you starve that they be better fed?' He then indeed starved – and re-fed – his volunteers, and in his classic 1950 book *The Biology of Starvation* he reported the preferential restocking of fat tissue on re-feeding. And though not all researchers, on repeating Keys's experiment, find the preferential restocking,[7] most do:[8] for once Keys told it like it probably is. Only if dieters consume a reasonable amount of protein – and take exercise – will they help sustain muscle mass.[9] My wife tells me, by the way, that this knowledge is widely known by personal trainers.

Resetting the metabolic and exercise rates: *The Biggest Loser* is an American reality television show where people compete to lose weight. Some people achieve massive weight loss (Danny Cahill, who is now 46, from Season 8, lost 239 pounds – 17 stones or 108 kg – in seven months) but, as the *New York Times* ran on its front page for 2 May 2016, these contestants then hit the problem of 'adaptive thermogenesis' (from the Greek *therme*, 'heat', and *gignesthai*, 'to be born'), which is a posh way of saying that human bodies will vary the amount of energy they use.

To be anthropomorphic, our bodies do not want to lose weight: our bodies are programmed by evolution to see starvation as a terrible threat, so a body that has experienced significant weight loss will, in a response that is sometimes known as the Survival of the Fattest, save energy by decreasing its metabolic rate. And that decrease may apparently be permanent. Nor are we talking small differences: in the words of an influential study: 'A formerly obese individual will require about 300–400 fewer calories per day to maintain the same body weight and physical activity level as a never-obese individual of the same body weight and composition.'[10]

The *Biggest Loser* research study from the National Institutes of Health, on which the *New York Times* based its story, found that the figure was higher, around 600 calories a day.[11] This number of calories is almost the size of a meal, and someone who's dieted will have to skip it permanently if they're to maintain the same weight as someone who's never dieted. Danny Cahill, for example, failed to do so, and he's now 104 pounds (7 stones 6 pounds, or 47 kg) heavier than he was seven years earlier.

Although some studies fail to find adaptive thermogenesis in dieters (which in the interests of balance I note here)[12], the majority do, and so we see how adaptive thermogenesis fights dieters. And, actually, it does so not only by slowing down their rate of metabolism but also by reducing the intensity of a phenomenon that is not widely recognised, namely casual exercise.

Physical activity can be monitored by portable meters or 'accelerometers' (the precursors of activity trackers such as Fitbits and Jawbones) and it transpires that dieters and post-dieters engage in less casual activity than their non-dieted peers: so dieters and post-dieters might take a lift rather than climb the stairs, or they might fidget less or drive short distances where once they would have walked.[13] Dieters and post-dieters seem, therefore, to lose the spontaneous impulse they once had to climb stairs or stretch their legs.

Adaptive thermogenesis thus offers another explanation for the paradox of breakfast skippers consuming few calories while being large: breakfast skippers will often be yo-yo dieters who (1) because of adaptive thermogenesis will burn relatively few calories, yet who (2) because of the yo-yo will be large. But it wasn't the breakfast skipping that enlarged these people, it was the yo-yo dieting-induced adaptive thermogenesis.

Hormones: Our hormones also don't want us to lose weight; a research group from Melbourne, Australia, found that overweight or obese subjects, on losing a significant amount of weight, demonstrate – even a year after the diet has stopped – higher levels of hormones such as ghrelin (which increases hunger) and lower levels of hormones such as leptin (which decreases hunger).[14]

Genes: Is our weight determined by our genes or our environment? Professor Tim Spector, the twin expert from King's College London, has found that: 'on average identical adult twins are less than 1 kg different in weight.'[15]

Genetics, in short, play a huge role (about two-thirds of the influence) in setting a person's weight,* and only about a third of the influence is due to the environment.[16] If we diet, therefore, in Professor Spector's words: 'Our bodies simply seem to adapt to the reduced calorie intake and do what they are programmed by evolution to do . . . This is why most diets fail.'[17]

Worryingly, weight-loss dieting might even induce weight *gain*. In 2012 a research group from Finland reported on identical twins where one of the twins had deliberately lost at least 5 kg (11 pounds, ¾ stone) on at least one occasion but where the other twin had

---

* To date some fifty-two so-called 'obesity genes' or variants have been linked with obesity, though no one variant in itself plays a strong role because, except for certain rare conditions, obesity and overweight are caused by combinations of genes interacting with our diets and rates of exercise (R.J. Loos (2011), 'Genetic determinants of common obesity and their value in prediction', *Best Pract Res Clin Endocrinol Metab* 26: 211–26). Though many of those genetic variants will act at the level of appetite control, some will act metabolically and others will help determine our portfolios of gut microbes.

never gone on a diet. And the dieters had eventually ended up, on average, 0.4 kg (1 pound) heavier than the non-dieters.[18]

Conclusion: A group from Switzerland, on reviewing the field, has concluded that slim people should never diet: they risk eventually putting on weight. Only large people should diet: only for them *might* it lead to weight loss.[19]

Dieting being unexpectedly problematic, we need to identify a strategy – a lifestyle – that allows people to lose weight *and* to keep it off. As we shall see, skipping breakfast will help achieve that.

8

Chaotic lives

There is another explanation for the apparent paradox of breakfast skippers being large: they may be leading chaotic lives. So a Finnish study of some 5,500 16-year-old girls and boys and their parents found that breakfast skippers tend to come from families that self-harm by:

- smoking
- failing to take sufficient exercise
- neglecting education
- consuming higher intakes of high-sugar, high-carbohydrate, high-fat snacks
- drinking too much
- being overweight.[1]

Extending those Finnish findings, a study from Rhode Island of nearly 10,000 adolescents showed a significant correlation between:

- breakfast skipping
- fast food eating
- weight gain.[2]

But correlation is not causation, so we need to ask, is it the breakfast skipping or the fast food eating that is causing the weight gain in these adolescents? Dr Mark Pereira of the University of Minnesota has answered that question. Dr Pereira followed 3,000 young adults over fifteen years, showing that those who ate at fast food restaurants more than twice a week gained an extra 10 pounds (4.5 kg), and had a twofold greater increase in insulin-resistance than those who ate there less than once a week.[3] Dr Pereira therefore confirmed that fast food is dangerous food, if only because it is so high in calories: 'a single meal from one of these restaurants often contains enough calories to satisfy a person's caloric requirements for an entire day.'[4]

And who eats fast food? People who lead chaotic lives. Dr Pereira divided his subjects into blacks and whites, and because – for shameful historical reasons – black Americans are disadvantaged, Dr Pereira thus also provided a link between social class and fast food. And Dr Pereira found that, fifteen years into the study:

- black people were visiting fast food restaurants 2.15 times a week against 1.60 times for white people
- the black people in Dr Pereira's study had nearly two years' less education than white people
- black people took three-quarters of the exercise of white people
- black people watched nearly twice as much television as white people
- black people ate some 400 calories more per day than white people
- black people drank 50 per cent more soft drinks than white people
- black people ate 50 per cent more meat than white people
- black people ate significantly less fibre than white people.

So the Rhode Island study on nearly 10,000 adolescents may have shown a significant correlation between breakfast skipping, fast food eating and weight gain, but from Dr Pereira's research we know it's not the breakfast skipping that is causing the weight gain, it's the fast food. And the fast food eating and the breakfast skipping have a common root in a chaotic lifestyle, so we can begin to see how breakfast skipping and overweight are not causally linked but, rather, reflect the actions of a separate, third, cause: domestic chaos leading to unhealthy life choices:

skip breakfast ➜ weight loss

smoke ➜ weight loss

➚

unhealthy lifestyle

➘

drink too much ➜ weight gain

too little exercise ➜ weight gain

eat too much ➜ weight gain

eat fattening food ➜ weight gain

whose net result is: ⚖ ➜ **weight gain**

So we can see how breakfast skipping may be *associated* with, but not *causative* of, weight gain. Breakfast skipping per se, in isolation, will promote weight loss, but if it is linked with a package of weight-gaining activities, it will then be associated with weight gain, thus leading unsuspecting epidemiologists to suppose that eating breakfast causes weight loss.

We might make a comparison with smoking and teenage pregnancy. Teenagers who smoke are more likely to become pregnant but no one has suggested that smoking causes pregnancy.[5] Rather, dysfunctional teenagers are more likely both to smoke and to become pregnant, but the causative agent is the dysfunction. Here is a model that captures that story:

➚ smoke

dysfunctional teenagers

➘ get pregnant

The model is *not*:

dysfunctional teenagers ➜ smoke ➜ get pregnant

And to confirm that model of association, not causation, there has even been a report that Japanese girls who skip breakfast also start to have sex two years before their breakfast-eating sisters (at 17.5 rather than 19.4 years of age). The report has not got into an English-language peer-reviewed journal, but it came from the Japan Family Planning Association, which is credible.[6] Here is a model that captures that story:

<pre>
                            ↗ skip breakfast
    dysfunctional teenagers
                            ↘ have premature sex
</pre>

The model is *not*:

dysfunctional teenagers → skip breakfast → have premature sex

---

Daniel, the lions' den and the earliest clinical trial

Epidemiology (from the Greek *epidamia*, the prevalence of disease) is the science of populations, but it's too easy in epidemiology to confuse cause and correlation. So here is a claim of cause:

eat breakfast → eat more → yet lose weight, paradoxically
(or alternatively)
skip breakfast → eat less → yet gain weight, paradoxically

and here is a claim of correlation:

<pre>
                        ↗ eat breakfast
        third factor
                        ↘ lose weight

    (or alternatively)
                        ↗ skip breakfast
        third factor
                        ↘ gain weight
</pre>

Epidemiological studies that look only at breakfast and weight can easily confuse correlation with cause – except that the science of epidemiology has long generated a 'hierarchy of evidence' by which to distinguish them, and it is a theme of this book that epidemiologists have not always been sufficiently rigorous in applying that hierarchy.

The hierarchy of evidence: Conflicts over diet are age-old, and some can be sourced to the Bible. Daniel was a Jew who had been captured by Nebuchadnezzar, the King of Babylon, and who was consequently condemned to various vicissitudes including the lions' den (from which, happily, he was rescued). Daniel was also instructed to eat the food of the royal court, to which he objected on grounds of observance. Let Daniel I: 12–16 take up the story of how he asked that he and his fellow captives be given:

> nothing but vegetables to eat and water to drink. Then [Daniel said] compare our appearance with that of the young men who eat the royal food, and treat your servants in accordance with what you see. So he [the chief official] agreed to this and tested them for ten days. At the end of the ten days they looked healthier and better nourished than any of the young men who ate the royal food. So the guard took away their choice food and the wine they were to drink and gave them vegetables instead [New International Version].

This was a clinical trial! The first to have been recorded. But though it wasn't too badly controlled, we think we can do better now, and today we understand that some methodologies are more powerful than others and that they can be ranked in a hierarchy of evidence:

- Systematic reviews and meta-analyses
- Randomised blinded controlled trials
- Randomised controlled trials
- Cohort studies
- Case-control studies
- Cross-sectional surveys
- Case reports.

Let me briefly look at these, starting with the weakest methodologies.[7]

7. Case reports: In such a report, the medical history of a patient is told as a story. 'Mr Joe Blogs has always smoked and he has just celebrated his eightieth birthday, therefore smoking potentiates longevity.' It doesn't require genius to understand why case reports provide only weak evidence of cause and effect.

6. Cross-sectional surveys: These are 'snapshots'. In such studies, people are asked two questions, which might be: what do you eat for breakfast and what is your weight? As I've shown above, many breakfast studies fall into this category, which is unfortunate because this sort of snapshot study can be very misleading, i.e. at any one time people may be large and thus skip breakfast while, later, those people may be slim and thus eat it, but it is not the eating of breakfast that makes you slim (and, vice versa, not the skipping of breakfast that makes you fat); rather, it's being large that encourages people to skip breakfast, and being slim that encourages people to eat it. So cross-sectional or snapshot studies can lead to conclusions that are 100 per cent wrong.

5. Case-control studies: These are not used frequently in breakfast research, so I'll not describe them here.

4. Cohort studies: These are an attempt at avoiding the problems of a 'snapshot'. In a cohort study, two groups of people are selected because they either do or do not eat breakfast (say) and then some years later their outcomes are determined. During the 1940s, 1950s and 1960s Bradford Hill and Richard Doll performed their famous cohort study on doctors who either did or did not smoke, discovering that smoking causes lung cancer.*

---

* Doll and Bradford published their ground-breaking paper in 1954, yet they had actually been scooped during the 1930s and 1940s by German scientists working to Hitler's anti-smoking agenda; but no one in the democracies was then very interested in Nazi science, and

3. Randomised controlled trials: Now we are moving from observations to experiments, where participants are given a drug or some other intervention (such as skipping breakfast or not eating the royal food) and scientists then determine the effect.

Experiments, though, are only as good as their controls: if you give a drug to a group of people and then get an effect, you need to know that those people were not going to produce that effect anyway, so in clinical medicine we do controlled trials, where the responses of subjects to a drug are compared to the responses of subjects who do not receive the drug. But the experimenter mustn't pick the control subjects, because that might bias the results, so in clinical medicine we do randomised controlled trials, where the two groups of subjects are selected to be as similar as possible, with individuals being distributed between the two groups randomly.

2. Randomised blinded controlled trials: Ideally, to avoid subconscious bias, neither the experimenters nor the subjects of a trial should know who is part of the intervention group and who is part of the control group, but unfortunately I need not explain this any further as we can't do blinded trials in breakfast: blinding requires that we provide control subjects with placebos, yet we can't provide placebos for breakfast. Breakfast studies have therefore been deprived of the most robust experimental protocols, but as the science of astronomy illustrates, knowledge can progress without the full panoply of experimental protocols: if we are careful in our observations, we can – in the absence of experiments – show that the earth moves round the sun rather than vice versa, but we do have to view the observations carefully, without preconceptions.

1. Systematic reviews and meta-analyses: These are sophisticated words that describe the sophisticated methods by which

---

the German research papers were simply ignored by the Anglophonic nations (R.N. Proctor (2012), 'The history of the discovery of the cigarette–lung cancer link: evidentiary traditions, corporate denial, global toll', *Tobacco Control* 21: 87–91).

the results of many different trials can be pooled, to provide more secure conclusions than any one trial can provide.

Conclusion: Clinical medicine has created a hierarchy of evidence, and in this book I try to show where breakfast epidemiologists have, unfortunately, ignored the hierarchy, to thus confuse correlation with cause.

———————————

9

Five breakfast sagas

I have explored the two major explanations for the apparent paradox of breakfast eaters consuming more calories than breakfast skippers while being slimmer; now let me offer five more:

1 Healthily minded people 'know' they should eat breakfast
2 People under-report their food intake
3 Breakfast skipping is not properly defined
4 'Kick-starting' metabolism
5 Breakfast skippers are owls, not larks.

Let's look at these in turn.

1. Healthily minded people 'know' they should eat breakfast (aka the 'compliance' effect): Consider a survey published in 2003 from the Massachusetts Medical School.[1] That survey confirmed that people who ate breakfast were slim, but the researchers warned that their 'findings cannot be considered causal' because most of their subjects were 'white middle class members of a health maintenance organization . . . [who] were highly motivated . . . in their own health'. And what in 2003 did members of health maintenance organisations know? They knew that breakfast was the most important meal of the day! Most of the survey's subjects were, therefore, complying with medical advice to eat breakfast, but they were also complying with the advice of not overeating during the course of the day.

Normally, of course, people do well to comply with medical advice, but such compliance can sometimes be dangerous. Consider vitamin D deficiency. A Swedish medical team has monitored a cohort of some 30,000 healthy women, of whom some 2,500 died from natural causes over twenty years. To minimise their risks of developing malignant melanoma, many of the women had avoided exposure to the sun. Such women had thus become vitamin D deficient and, as a consequence, their overall death rate from all disease . . . doubled. In the words of the paper: 'the mortality rate amongst avoiders of sun exposure was approximately twofold higher compared with the highest sun exposure group . . . the effect was presumably attributable to cancer, heart disease and cerebrovascular disease.'[2]

Compliance dangers are perennial because medical science advances perennially, and such advances invariably take doctors and patients into unknown territory, where the law of unintended consequences can apply. And one important compliance danger is breakfast. Your doctor may assure you that breakfast is the most important meal of the day, but that self-same doctor would once have assured you that babies have to be laid to sleep on their tummies (see below).

Cot deaths and neonatal blindness: compliance dangers

When our first child was born, in 1991, the world was still in the grip of the epidemic of cot deaths that had, unexpectedly, erupted some years earlier. To minimise the risks to our child, my wife and I were told to lay her to sleep on her tummy. But when our second child was born, in 1993, we were told to lay him on his back. It transpired that more than half of cot deaths before 1992 had occurred because babies had been laid to sleep on their tummies; and they were sleeping on their tummies because studies had shown that sick babies in intensive care units did better on their tummies.

Fair enough. But that observation was then extrapolated, without proper testing, to healthy babies at home; and those do *worse* on their tummies, so their death rates rose.[3]

Perhaps the best-known example of compliance danger is provided by Stevie Wonder, whose blindness was caused by his having been given, as a sick baby, 100 per cent oxygen to breathe. Routinely giving 100 per cent oxygen to sick babies – regardless of their illness and regardless of their actual need for extra oxygen – was once conventional until doctors realised that the contemporary epidemic of infant blindness was being caused by the excessive oxygen that, by stimulating the uncontrolled growth of certain cells in the eyes, was destroying the babies' vision.

We can go on multiplying the recent examples of doctors being wrong (I'm not talking leeches here, I'm talking about modern doctors). Consider hormone replacement therapy (HRT) for the menopause. For half a century this was lauded by doctors, and for years 'it was considered malpractice if you did not prescribe HRT for menopausal women.'[4] Only with the publication of the two Women's Health Initiatives in 1992 did the breast cancer story emerge, and HRT is now prescribed with circumspection.[5]

These stories are relevant to breakfast because they confirm that modern doctors can sometimes be wrong in their advice, advice over breakfast not excluded.

---

2. People under-report their food intake: Another breakfast confounder is that obese people tend to under-report their food intake, so the association between obesity and breakfast skipping may be simply a reporting artefact: obese people may be eating breakfast, and thus getting fat, but they may be reporting themselves as not eating breakfast.[6]

I have no doubt that large people, like most people actually, under-report their eating, though large people may be particularly extreme under-reporters. In the days when, as a young doctor, I ran metabolic clinics, I would be astonished by the vehemence with which some overweight and obese patients denied the obvious fact that they ate excessively. I remember one very large lady who denied eating between meals, whose daughter approached me discreetly to say that her mother ate biscuits all day, claiming 'they didn't count.'

3. Breakfast skipping is not properly defined: In 2008 a philosopher, Peter Vranas of the University of Wisconsin, noted that different research groups were using up to twenty-four different definitions of breakfast skipping. These ranged from never consuming a calorie before midday, to never consuming one before 10.00 a.m., to consuming a light drink of milk or fruit juice on occasion or regularly, to eating a full breakfast but only at weekends, etc., etc. And Vranas found ... well, let the title of his paper speak for itself: 'Breakfast skipping and body mass index among adolescents in Greece: whether an association exists depends on how breakfast skipping is defined'.[7]

This was an alarming finding because it suggested that different research groups had published different conclusions based solely on different definitions of breakfast skipping.

Vranas has shown, in short, that much of the epidemiological literature may have been distorted by loose definitions. We probably need more philosophers in this area.

4. 'Kick-starting' metabolism: On eating a meal, a person's metabolic rate increases as they consume energy in digesting the food (which is why some people feel hot or sweaty during or after a meal). So a number of researchers have suggested that if (*if!*) the eating of breakfast is slimming, perhaps that is because eating breakfast stimulates metabolism all day long, thus burning calories all day long. That suggestion is echoed commercially: easyJet's on-board magazine *Bistro & Boutique* for March 2015 carried a claim from the CEO of Moma, a porridge company, saying that breakfast 'kick starts your metabolism'.[8]

But in 2014 a research team led by James Betts from the

University of Bath, UK, performed the most comprehensive study to date.[9] Studying a group of subjects over six weeks, half of whom ate breakfast and half of whom did not, Betts first confirmed that breakfast satiety is a myth: when his subjects ate breakfast they consumed 539 extra calories overall during the day (i.e. skippers consumed 539 fewer calories overall). But then he found that, after six weeks of daily breakfast, 'contrary to popular belief there was no . . . increased resting metabol-ism': i.e. he'd exploded the myth that breakfast kick-started metabolism. Dr Betts went on to tell the *Daily Mail*:

> The belief that breakfast is 'the most important meal of the day' is so widespread that many people are surprised to learn that there is a lack of scientific evidence showing whether or how breakfast may directly cause changes in our health. It is certainly true that people who regularly eat breakfast tend to be slimmer and healthier but these individuals also typically follow most other recommendations for a healthy lifestyle, so have more balanced diets and take more physical exercise.[10]

Indeed, in a similar study on obese people, Betts concluded that: 'In view of the public perception that breakfast consumption facilitates weight management, it is paradoxical that 10 of the 11 individuals in the breakfast group gained weight.'[11]

As Betts told the *Independent* on 24 March 2016, breakfast 'is not going to make you lose weight' so there's no need to hypothesise a mythical metabolic kick-start to account for a mythical weight loss. There's no *if*.

And Betts himself – a man who knows more about breakfast than most of us – generally skips it.

5. Breakfast skippers are owls, not larks: A recent study from Finland on over 6,000 people showed that evening types were two and a half times more likely to develop type 2 diabetes than were morning types.[12] That dramatic finding is signifi-cant because a separate study has shown that evening types often skip breakfast.[13] These two studies thus provide a strong correlation between breakfast skipping and the development of type 2 diabetes, but the underlying cause appears to be so-called 'social jet lag'.

Evening types or owls seem to suffer from social jet lag because, having gone to bed late, they are always having to wake earlier than they would like. These owls compensate for tiredness or 'sleep debt' during the week by lying in over the weekend, but in the meantime they suffer from stress and depression. So, for example, one study from Munich, reporting on some 500 volunteers, discovered that the more someone was an owl, the more likely they were to smoke and drink excessively.[14]

Equally, another study from Chicago and Bangkok, reporting on patients with type 2 diabetes, showed that the more a person was an owl (which was determined by how much extra sleep they took – and by how late they got up – at weekends) the more likely they were to skip breakfast and the more likely they were to be overweight and to have severe diabetes. They were also more likely to develop hypertension.[15]

These studies showed, therefore, that the breakfast skipping of social jet lag was – like the smoking and drinking and stress and depression and obesity and diabetes of social jet lag – just one of the complications of the social jet lag: the skipping did not cause the complications, it was one more to add to the list.[16]

The damage caused by social jet lag is mediated by sleep deprivation, but social jet lag is, of course, not the only cause of sleep deprivation, and a research group from Okayama, Japan, has shown that people who have difficulty in getting to sleep for whatever reason, or who wake up at night for whatever reason, are also two and a half times more likely to develop type 2 diabetes.[17] And a recent study from Sweden on healthy young men who were kept awake artificially showed that on the following day they ate significantly more food.[18]

Sleep deprivation also damages by raising the levels of stress compounds in the blood including cortisol, certain pro-inflammatory chemicals and free fatty acids.[19] These promote insulin-resistance and thus obesity and type 2 diabetes.[20]

From all these different studies, therefore, it appears that:

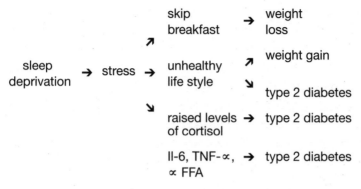

whose net result is: ⚖ → **weight gain + type 2 diabetes**

So we have uncovered yet one more association between breakfast skipping, obesity and diabetes which owes nothing to cause and effect but which, rather, is rooted in a common factor of sleep deprivation.*

Finally, a good Darwinian would be compelled to find a compensatory benefit to being an owl: if owls are less healthy than larks, they should surely have gone extinct by now, yet it has been reported that night owls are more intelligent than morning larks, which perhaps explains their survival.[21]

---

* Famously, Winston Churchill went to bed very late indeed, but – equally famously – he catnapped during the day, and in so doing he may have anticipated recent developments in endocrinology. When a Paris research group restricted eleven healthy young men to only two hours' sleep a night, the subjects' levels of norepinephrine (which is a hormone that raises blood glucose levels) and of interleukin-6 (which is a chemical that promotes inflammation) both rose. But on catnapping during the day, the young men could reverse their unhealthy hormonal responses (B Faraut et al. (10 February 2015), 'Napping reverses the salivary interleukin-6 and urinary norepinephrine changes induced by sleep restriction', *Journal of Clinical Endocrinology and Metabolism*, doi: http://dx.doi.org/10.1210/jc.2014-2566). It is perhaps no coincidence that the catnapping Churchill lived to be 90, though that is only a case report.

Recent (welcome) developments: As we increasingly understand the links between breakfast skipping and obesity to be
an association, not causation, it's good to report that scientists
are, today, increasingly careful not to conflate them. So, for
example, a 2010 overview of sixteen different European studies
that found breakfast skipping and obesity to be linked nonetheless concluded that since 'almost all of the data . . . were
gathered from observational studies . . . causality should not
be assumed'.[22] Epidemiological sanity is beginning to win out.

Much breakfast epidemiology has only confirmed what
Michael Marmot from University College London established
long ago, namely that in the west the upper socio-economic
groups outlive the lower groups by about seven years, probably because they experience less stress.* And since the upper
socio-economic groups tend to comply with the conventional
advice to eat breakfast and other regular meals, while the lower
groups tend to eat less regularly, much epidemiology reflects
only a correlation between frequent eating and longevity.

---

* M.G. Marmot et al. (1997), 'Contribution of job control and other
risk factors to social variations in heart disease incidence', *Lancet* 350:
235–9.

PART FIVE

Breakfast Wars

The two most distinguished universities
on the planet, Harvard and Cambridge,
continue to promote breakfast as healthy,
but heroic guerrillas from Cornell and
Alabama are confronting them.

10

The Harvard and Cambridge challenges

Harvard has for years been studying the 51,529 middle-aged professional white men of the Health Professionals Follow-Up Study (HPFS). These men were recruited in 1992, and it happened that some 17 per cent of them were breakfast skippers, which is a typical percentage.

At least three important breakfast-related findings concerning weight gain, type 2 diabetes and coronary heart disease have apparently come out of this politically incorrect Follow-Up Study on middle-aged upper middle-class white men:

- In 2007 the scientists of the HPFS reported that 'the consumption of breakfast may modestly contribute to the prevention of *weight gain* compared with skipping breakfast in middle-aged and older men' [1]
- In 2012 the scientists reported that 'breakfast omission was associated with an increased risk of *type 2 diabetes*' [2]
- And in 2013 the scientists reported that 'eating breakfast was associated with significantly lower *coronary heart disease* risk in this cohort of male health professionals' [3] [all my italics].

But we would be hasty to accept the associations as causations. First, the breakfast skippers are unquestionably following risky lifestyles: men who skipped breakfast smoked three times more, exercised less, drank more coffee and alcohol, and ate significantly less healthy foods than men who ate breakfast. Breakfast skippers were also 21 per cent more likely to snack, were a bit fatter, and were more likely to eat late at night. In the 2013 coronary heart study, moreover, the researchers also found that breakfast eaters were more likely to be married (marriage is good for men's health)* and that skippers were significantly less likely to get regular health check-ups.

In their three breakfast studies, the Harvard scientists of the HPFS tried to correct statistically for those confounding factors, but I suspect they failed to do so – not because they didn't try hard enough but because there are simply too many unknown factors. So, for example, no correction was made for social support (people with good networks of friends tend to live longer than the friendless,[4] and they also tend to eat breakfast,[5] which does *not* tell us that eating breakfast is a good way of keeping friends, nor that eating breakfast is healthy, but rather that compliance with conventional human norms such as friendship

---

* A Framingham survey of 3,682 people showed that over a three-year period married men were 46 per cent less likely than unmarried men to die (E.D. Eaker et al. (2007), 'Marital status, marital strain, and risk of coronary heart disease or total mortality: the Framingham Offspring Study', *Psychosom Med* 69: 509–13). But only monogamous marriage is good for men's health: a preliminary study on 687 married men in Saudi Arabia showed that the more wives a man had, the more likely he was to suffer from coronary artery disease; 68 per cent of those 687 men had one wife, 19 per cent had two, 10 per cent had three, and 3 per cent had four wives, and the study found that polygamy raised the risk of developing coronary artery disease 4.6-fold. The really shocking statistic to emerge from the Saudi study, though, was that 56 per cent of the men, whose average age was 59 years, had diabetes; 57 per cent, moreover, had hypertension and 45 per cent had a history of coronary artery disease (A. Daoulah (2015), as reported by www.escardio.org/The-ESC/Press-releases/Last-5-years/Polygamy-increases-risk-of-heart-disease-by-more-than-4-fold). The insulin-resistance of type 2 diabetes and the metabolic syndrome are apparently epidemic if not pandemic in Saudi Arabia.

leads to better health outcomes, even if certain aspects of that compliance – *viz* breakfast – are unhealthy).* Until correction has been made for the full panoply of risks, we simply cannot accept Harvard's claims that breakfast is safe.

Moreover, the HPFS scientists have finally confirmed that the satiety hypothesis has been disproved, and in their 2013 paper they reported that breakfast eaters consumed 123 calories a day more than the skippers. Cumulatively, this should lead to the breakfast eaters putting on a pound of fat (0.5 kg) more, every month, than the skippers, so Harvard's own data suggest that breakfast is unhealthy.

Yet the Harvard HPFS researchers remain wedded to breakfast being healthy as a cause-and-effect paradigm. So though in 2013 they wrote, very properly, that 'it is possible that eating habits could be a marker of lifestyle consistency or general health-seeking behaviour', they seem not to really believe in correlation. So in 2007, for example, before they recognised that breakfast eaters ate more calories, they wrote: 'The prevalence of overweight and obesity has rapidly increased in recent decades . . . The prevalence of people not consuming breakfast every day has increased over the last decades . . . Breakfast consumption could reduce total calorific intake during the day by consuming less food during the day,'[6] which was a clear statement of the linear breakfast paradigm of:

eat breakfast ➔ satiety ➔ consume ➔ lose weight
less food

or vice versa

skip breakfast ➔ no satiety ➔ consume ➔ increase weight
more food

---

* Fruit and vegetable intake are markedly associated with good social support (A. Mirzaei et al. (2016), 'Social cognitive predictors of breakfast consumption in primary school's male students', *Globl J Health Sci* 8: 124–32).

And though the Harvard scientists have since had to shed that particular cause-and-effect paradigm, they seem to have adopted stress as a cause instead. Dr Leah Cahill was the lead author of the 2013 HPFS coronary heart disease study, and she revealed what she believes to reporters from Texas A&M University's newsletter and *Forbes* magazine, who wrote that: 'Cahill says that fasting is a stressful state for the body, so prolonging the fast by not eating when you wake up amplifies the stress.'[7]

Dr Cahill repeated the same message when she spoke to the BBC, saying that skipping breakfast and so not 'breaking fast' put extra strain on the body.[8] But I can find no actual evidence from Harvard showing skipping breakfast to be stressful.

Indeed, another clue that the successive HPFS studies do not provide the final word on breakfast was shown by their contradictory results over eating frequency: their different studies could not agree on the optimal numbers of meals to be eaten daily:

i   In 2007 (the weight gain study) the HPFS scientists reported that 'an *increasing* number of eating occasions . . . was associated with a higher risk of 5-kg weight gain'

ii In 2009 (the type 2 study) they reported that 'compared with men who ate 3 times a day, men who ate 1–2 times a day had a higher risk of type 2 diabetes' (i.e. a *decreasing* number of eating occasions was associated with a higher risk of type 2)

iii And in 2013 (the coronary heart disease study) they reported that '*No* association was observed between eating frequency . . . and risk of coronary heart disease' (all my italics).

Since breakfast skipping is itself a variation in meal frequency, these contradictory findings suggest not that breakfast skipping leads to weight gain, diabetes and coronary heart disease but, rather, that a separate set of factors leads both to breakfast skipping and to the diseases.

Cambridge UK: Harvard is situated in Cambridge, MA, but the scientists in Cambridge UK are also fans of breakfast. In one study the Cambridge epidemiologists wanted to know how breakfast determined weight gain, so they performed a cross-sectional or 'snapshot' study. They recruited some 6,800 middle-aged men and women, some of whom, of course, happened to eat light breakfasts, while others happened to eat big ones.[9]

The research team asked their subjects (i) what they typically ate for breakfast, and (ii) what else they typically ate during the course of the day. The research team then weighed them, finding that the more food they ate at breakfast, the more calories overall they consumed, yet the lighter they weighed, i.e.:

eat breakfast ➔ consume more calories ➔ weigh less ???

The research team had apparently, therefore, reaffirmed the (in)famous breakfast paradox: the team had confirmed that satiety is a myth (the more the subjects ate at breakfast, the more they ate overall), but since the breakfast eaters were slimmer than the skippers, the paradox had apparently re-emerged. But paradoxes emerge only when a false paradigm hits reality, so which paradigm were the researchers working to? Here is an extract from the introduction to their paper: '[Studies show that] regular breakfast consumption is associated with successful maintenance of weight loss, suggesting that consuming fewer calories in the morning or skipping breakfast could contribute to the development of obesity.'

So the researchers were working to a cause-and-effect paradigm:

eat breakfast ➔ eat more food overall ➔ lose weight
or
skip breakfast ➔ eat less food overall ➔ gain weight

which makes no sense. But if we adopt a different paradigm:

No history of dieting, therefore brisk metabolism
↓
therefore can afford to eat breakfast
↓
yet still lose weight

or alternatively:

History of dieting, therefore slow metabolism
↓
therefore cannot afford to eat breakfast
↓
yet still gain weight

then we have a model that is not paradoxical. So if we rewrite the introduction to the paper, we can keep the first half of the sentence, which contains the facts, but we can change the conclusion: '[Studies show that] regular breakfast consumption is associated with successful maintenance of weight loss, suggesting that *slim people can afford to eat breakfast and to consume more calories.*'

The Cambridge researchers then reinforced their observations by performing a cohort study analogous to the one Hill and Doll performed on smokers. They followed their subjects over the next 3.7 years, finding that on average:

- all their subjects gained weight as they aged
- the people who ate the lightest breakfasts gained some 1.25 kg
- those who ate the biggest breakfasts gained only some 0.8 kg
- even though they apparently consumed, on average, 82 calories a day more than the small breakfast eaters.

Yet again, the researchers had apparently uncovered the (in)famous paradox. But they then did an odd thing. They interpreted their findings to conclude that the 'redistribution of daily energy intake, so that a larger percentage is consumed at breakfast and a lower percentage is consumed over the rest of the day, may help to reduce weight gain in middle-aged adults.'

Yet that is *not* the full conclusion of the paper's own logic or data: the researchers showed that the more breakfast their subjects ate, the more food they also ate. So using the researchers' own logic and their own data, the full conclusion is: 'To keep slim, eat more at breakfast, and ensure your total food intake also goes up.' Which makes no sense, which is why I assume the Cambridge scientists didn't draw the logical conclusion of their own data.

Cambridge and Dr Farshchi: The Cambridge scientists knew their findings were paradoxical, so to explain them they invoked the work of Dr Farshchi, from the University of Nottingham.

Dr Farshchi was a researcher who had examined the insulin responses of ten women, finding that when they skipped breakfast, their circulating levels of insulin rose (and vice versa, the levels of insulin in breakfast eaters fell).[10] Since insulin makes you fat, the Cambridge researchers suggested, the paradox was therefore solved:

skip breakfast ➜ secrete more insulin ➜ get fat
or
eat breakfast ➜ secrete less insulin ➜ stay slim

Hold on. Eat breakfast and secrete *less* insulin? Skip breakfast and secrete *more*? The whole point of insulin is that it rises when we eat (I discuss this at greater length later), so what's happening when the more that people eat, the less insulin they secrete?

Well, it turns out that when Dr Farshchi's subjects ate breakfast, they ingested less food overall. And vice versa: when they skipped breakfast they ate more overall. They were anomalous. This was something that Dr Farshchi signposted himself, writing that his findings were 'at variance with previous stud-ies'. (The previous studies show, of course, that breakfast eaters, like the Cambridge team's subjects, consume more calories.)

So Dr Farshchi's findings *cannot* resolve the Cambridge researchers' paradox, because the Cambridge team's breakfast eaters ingested *more* food overall whereas Dr Farshchi's break-fast eaters ingested *less*.

I hope I have not been unfair to the Cambridge scientists, whose papers are, rightly, widely read, and whose data can be trusted unreservedly, and who are scrupulously honest, but we do need to know if eating breakfast is good or bad for us, and if we adopt their paradox we have to conclude (in my summary of their logic) that:

> to keep slim, eat more at breakfast and ensure your total
> food intake also goes up

whereas if we refuse to accept a paradox, then the data suggest that:

> to keep slim, skip breakfast, which will lower your total
> food intake.

The choice is black or white, but the consequences may be life or premature death.

And though I totally respect the Cambridge scientists' data, I do regret one set of facts they seem to have omitted: they appear to have excluded from their analysis all the subjects who died or fell ill over the 3.7 years they monitored them. But it is a principle in epidemiology that the most important poten-tial end-point of an investigation is not a proxy measurement (such as obesity) but the end-point itself, namely death. The team might still have those data, and it would be good to see them published. Do they show if breakfast kills or cures?

Why were Dr Farshchi's subjects anomalous?

Why were Dr Farshchi's breakfast eaters eating less, overall, than the breakfast skippers? Or, to rephrase the question, why were the breakfast skippers eating more, overall, than the breakfast eaters?

Well, Dr Farshchi studied only ten women, whom we have to conclude were simply unrepresentative of the wider population. Different people can respond dramatically differently to the same food. Consider blood glucose. In 2015 two Israeli scientists published a comprehensive study on no fewer than 800 people, finding that 'people eating identical meals present high variability in post-meal blood glucose responses.'[11]

Consider bread. There is a *ninefold difference* between different people's blood sugar responses to breakfast bread, with some people registering only a pimple on the graph while others register a huge rise. Some people, remarkably, register higher levels of blood glucose after eating bread than after eating the equivalent amount of glucose itself. In some people, moreover, bananas raise blood glucose levels worryingly but cookies are completely safe, yet for other people the exact reverse is true. And for some people tomatoes are dangerous.

These variabilities should not have been surprising: in a classic experiment from 1990, a Quebec study isolated twelve pairs of young male twins, and for four months overfed all twenty-four men by 1,000 calories a day, almost as if they were geese on a *pâté de fois gras* production line. On average, the men gained 8.1 kg (18 pounds or 1¼ stones) but the range was considerable, from 4.3 kg to 13.3 kg.[12] Intriguingly, though, each twin gained almost the same amount of weight as their fellow twin; i.e. different people's metabolisms are very different indeed, and the differences are largely genetic.

People, in short, have inherited very different responses to food, so nutritional studies on only ten people will inevitably be overwhelmed by individuals' quirks. Indeed, a later breakfast experiment by Dr Farshchi's colleagues in Nottingham on twelve men found

that the 'combined energy intake [breakfast and lunch] did not differ between the breakfast and no-breakfast trials',[13] i.e., when those
Nottingham scientists repeated their own experiment on twelve
men, they got different results from when they'd performed it on
ten women – with both sets of findings being at variance with previous studies. To get a solid breakfast finding, therefore, it may not
be necessary to study 800 folk the way Segal and Elinav did, but
equally we must view findings on ten or twelve subjects as only
preliminary and potentially misleading, not definitive.

It was scrupulously honest of Dr Farshchi to admit to the anomalous nature of his experiment, but it is nonetheless depressing that
his paper has been cited over 200 times (including by the Harvard
scientists), and though I've not checked every paper that has cited
it, every one I have checked has cited it to confirm a breakfast
hypothesis that the data in the paper actually disprove. Dismaying.

11

The heroic breakfast guerrillas

It takes courage to flout the dominant paradigm, so let me here signpost the work of a small group of brave resisters.

David Allison: In 2013 David Allison and his colleagues from the University of Alabama at Birmingham reviewed ninety-two studies known to have reported on skipping breakfast. Their review had a dramatic title, 'Belief beyond the evidence: Using the proposed effect of breakfast on obesity to show 2 practices that distort scientific evidence', but their review lived up to the billing, showing that breakfast researchers regularly misrepresent not only their own results but also those of other researchers. So, for example, Allison reported that no fewer than 62 per cent of the papers he surveyed cited just one particular study in a 'misleading' fashion. Allison concluded that: 'The scientific record is distorted by research lacking probative value and biased research reporting.'[1]

This conclusion was challenged by researchers from Harvard University's School of Public Health, who argued that Allison had not disproved the suggestion that breakfast skipping caused obesity;[2] to which Allison responded by saying he was not trying to disprove it, he was showing that no one had actually established the causation in the first place.[3]

In 2014, moreover, in a randomised controlled trial, Allison divided obese or overweight adults into three weight-loss groups, who either

- ate breakfast every day
- ate no breakfasts
- ate however they wanted.

And after sixteen weeks there was no difference in weight between the three groups.[4]

In so doing Allison replicated a 1992 study from Nashville, Tennessee, which reported that when moderately obese women were put on identical weight-reduction diets, differing only in the provision or otherwise of breakfast (the breakfast skippers ate more at lunch and dinner to compensate for the skipped calories) there was no difference in the rate of weight loss.[5]

David Levitsky: It's not only southerners who are seceding from the dominant paradigm. On 1 August 2014 David Levitsky of Cornell University, NY, wrote an editorial for the *American Journal of Clinical Nutrition* declaring war on breakfast. It was Levitsky who, with Carly Pacanowski, had shown (above) that breakfast does not induce satiety – rather, it increases food consumption – so Levitsky has been a pioneer in exploding breakfast myths. This is how he opened his editorial:

> Three articles appear in this issue of the Journal that challenge
> a long-held belief of both nutrition scientists and the lay public:
> breakfast is the most important meal of the day. Of course
> this is true, if you are selling breakfast cereals. Putting profits
> aside, the consumption of breakfast is currently part of
> 1) most weight-reduction procedures and 2) school breakfast
> programs designed to improve cognitive/school performance.
> The publication of these articles may give us reason to
> examine the veracity of these ideas.[6]

This is not a paragraph that needs translating into ordinary English. Nor does the last paragraph of the editorial need translating:

Myths abound in nutrition. Many, like the consumption of breakfast, are driven by powerful commercial interests. In the current environment in which the major nutritional problem we face is the increasing prevalence of obesity, we, as nutrition scientists, must consider the possible harm we are doing by perpetuating myths such as the value of consuming breakfast.

Recent (welcome) developments: Allison and Levitsky are not the only scientists to have challenged Harvard's approach to epidemiology. Here are four recent *Times* headlines:

- Daily yoghurt may cut risk of diabetes[7]
- Daily bowl of porridge is key to longer life[8]
- Eat a few peanuts a day to slash risk of early death[9]
- Biggest-ever study proves berries and grapes help weight loss[10]

All four studies came from Harvard or Harvard collaborators, and though each paper invariably contained formal warnings that the findings were only associations, the tone of the papers nonetheless justified *The Times*'s cheerleading headlines.

But *The Times* also collated some robust responses:

- 'It could be that those eating yoghurt were more likely to lead a healthy lifestyle' (Alastair Rankin, the director of Diabetes UK, 14 November 2014)
- 'People with a higher intake of whole grains also tend to have a healthier overall lifestyle and diet' (Victoria Taylor, senior dietician at the British Heart Foundation, 6 January 2015)
- 'We know that in this study peanut eaters were leaner, ate more fruits and vegetables . . . were less likely to have high blood pressure or diabetes . . . these factors combined are a more powerful influence on mortality than a nibble of peanuts daily' (Catherine Collins, the senior dietician at St George's Hospital, London, 11 June 2015)

- 'This type of study cannot prove a cause-and-effect . . . individuals who eat more high-flavonoid foods have other habits which lead them to put on less weight' (Professor Sattar of the University of Glasgow, 26 January 2016).

We seem to be witnessing a healthy tendency in dietary epidemiology by which those researchers who are prone to believing in linear or causative relationships, including over breakfast, are being increasingly challenged by those who acknowledge correlation. And some people now worry that Harvard is insufficiently concerned with publishing the facts as they fall out of the observations; rather, people worry, Harvard is too concerned about the consistency of its public health messages.[11]

And this scepticism is now spilling over, publicly, into breakfast. The US government's *2010–2015 Dietary Guidelines for Americans* stated that 'not eating breakfast has been associated with excess body weight,'[12] which was a strong anti-skipping nudge, yet in a story in the *Washington Post* of 10 August 2015 entitled 'The science of skipping breakfast: How government nutritionists may have gotten it wrong', the journalist Peter Whoriskey argued that the nudge was not based on science but on speculation. In Whoriskey's damning sentence: 'A closer look at the way the government nutritionists adopted the breakfast warning for the *Dietary Guidelines* shows how loose scientific guesses – possibly right, possibly wrong – can be elevated into hard-and-fast federal nutrition rules that are broadcast throughout the United States.'

As Whoriskey pointed out, the epidemiological studies that recommend breakfast are only observational, and he quoted S. Stanley Young, the former director of bioinformatics at the National Institute of Statistical Sciences, who said, 'Wow. Is this really science? Every observational study could be challenged.'[13]

PART SIX

Misleading Experiments

I hope I've persuaded you that most of
the epidemiology of breakfast is flawed,
and in Part 6 I shall show the same
of the biochemistry.

12

Blood glucose and breakfast:
the unhealthy majority

In Chapter 1 I reported how both Professor Christiansen and I had found that blood glucose levels rose disproportionately after breakfast in type 2 diabetics, and that – because raised levels of blood glucose are dangerous – breakfast was in consequence an unusually dangerous meal for those patients. Simultaneous discovery is a feature in science* (famously, Charles Darwin had to rush his *Origin of Species* into print in 1859 after Alfred Russel Wallace had had the same insight into evolution by natural selection) so, equally, this type 2 diabetic breakfast discovery has been made independently by at least four other research groups.

Rather than force the reader to plough through all the papers, I've collated them in the box on the next page.

---

* In his perceptive 2015 book *The Evolution of Everything* Matt Ridley describes how simultaneous discovery is – contrary to myth – the norm in science and technology. According to Ridley, the scientists' and technologists' obsession with priority, prizes and patents is excessive and often unfair.

Blood glucose levels after breakfast in type 2 diabetes

- in 2009 Dr Raj Peter and his colleagues from the Diabetes Research Unit, Penarth, UK, studied forty-nine patients with type 2 diabetes. Though he fed them the same meals at breakfast, lunch and dinner, breakfast increased their circulating blood glucose levels by 35 per cent more than did lunch or dinner. Dr Peter thus confirmed that, for type 2 diabetics, lunch and dinner were the most important meals of the day; breakfast was dangerous[1]

- in a study on 248 patients with type 2 diabetes, a Montpelier/Swansea research collaboration gave their subjects only half as many calories at breakfast than at lunch or dinner, yet 'the highest peak glucose value . . . was observed in the post-breakfast period'.[2] And we are not talking small differences: breakfast, though containing only half as much food as either lunch or dinner, drove blood glucose levels 40 per cent higher from baseline

- and in 2013 Dr Hans Guldbrand and his colleagues from the department of medicine in Linkoping, Sweden, found that if type 2 diabetics skipped breakfast and, instead, bundled it into a large lunch, their post-lunch blood glucose levels were no higher than if they had eaten only a normal lunch, thus confirming that lunch was, for type 2 diabetics, a safer meal than breakfast[3]

- finally, in 1996, Dr Guenther Boden and his colleagues from the Temple University School of Medicine, Philadelphia, on studying six type 2 diabetics, found that in the morning their livers pour glucose into the bloodstream. Dr Boden's 'results are compatible with a large body of evidence showing [that] in patients with non-insulin dependent diabetes . . . plasma glucose levels rise in the early morning hours'.[4]

Clearly, therefore, to eat breakfast and thus further raise blood glucose levels when they are naturally at their highest *must* be dangerous for these patients.

Further, there are two conditions that are closely associated with type 2 diabetes, namely prediabetes and obesity, and these patients' blood glucose levels after breakfast confirm that, for them too, breakfast is a dangerous meal (see below).

Blood glucose levels after breakfast in prediabetes and obesity

- in 2006 Dr Maria dos Santos and her colleagues from the University of São Paulo, Brazil, on studying fifteen subjects with prediabetes, found their blood glucose levels after breakfast were higher than after lunch or dinner, even though they ate only half as much at breakfast than at the other two meals[5]

- and in 1988 Dr Polonsky of the University of Chicago, on studying fifteen obese people, found that if he gave them only half as many calories at breakfast than at lunch, their glucose levels nonetheless rose nearly twice as much, thus showing that breakfast was clearly a dangerous meal for them.[6]

But just as it seemed that breakfast had been confirmed to be dangerous in type 2 diabetes and its associated conditions, two studies were published in 2015 apparently showing the opposite. They were published jointly by Professors Daniela Jakubowicz (Tel Aviv University) and Oren Froy (Hebrew University of Jerusalem). The message of their first paper[7] was reported, accurately, on 25 February 2015 by *The Times* in its headline: 'Diabetics better off with high-energy breakfast'.

That was a startling message yet, oddly, the study does *not* show breakfast to be a safe meal. In fact, its breakfast findings are indistinguishable from Professor Christiansen's. So, on studying eighteen middle-aged type 2 diabetics, Professors Jakubowicz and Froy found that, like Professor Christiansen's patients, they woke in the mornings with high blood glucose levels, at around 7 mmol/l, and that when they ate a breakfast of 700 calories, their blood glucose levels rose even higher than Professor Christiansen's. So Professors Jakubowicz and Froy had actually confirmed that, for type 2 diabetics, breakfast is a dangerous meal. So how did their paper turn into a story of breakfast safety?

Well, let's look at their other 2015 paper,[8] whose message was accurately summarised by Tel Aviv University on its website: 'Diabetics who skip breakfast provoke hazardous blood sugar spikes.'[9] The website continued:

> The clinical study was conducted on 22 type-2 diabetics who averaged 56.0 years old, with a mean Body Mass Index of 28.2 kg/m^2 [i.e. they were overweight]. Over the course of two days, the participants consumed precisely the same numbers of calories and the same balanced meal – milk, tuna, bread, and a chocolate breakfast bar – for lunch and dinner. The only difference was that one day they ate breakfast and the second day they fasted until lunch. 'We theorized that the omission of breakfast would not be healthy, but it was surprising to see the high degree of deterioration of glucose metabolism only because the participants did not eat breakfast,' said Prof. Jakubowicz. The researchers found that participants experienced extraordinary glucose peaks of 268mg/dl (14.8 mmol/l) after lunch and 298mg/dl (16.5 mmol/l) after dinner on days they skipped breakfast, versus only 192 mg/dl (10.6 mmol/l), and 215 mg/dl (11.9 mmol/l) after eating an identical lunch and dinner on days they ate breakfast.

That looks pretty damning of skipping breakfast, but there are three points about the professors' own university website report that are wrong. First, the figures are incorrect. Actually, the participants' glucose peaks at dinner on the days they ate breakfast were 236, not 215 mg/dl, so the differences between the breakfast-skipping and breakfast-eating days were not so extraordinary (298 against 236). Less grievously, but still odd, the website also reported the figure for the breakfast-skipping dinners incorrectly (298 v 294 mg/dl).

Second, the website said that the experiments were performed 'over the course of two days' but, actually, they were performed over the course of six days. This is important because of the third error, which was contained within the quote from Professor Jakubowicz: 'it was surprising to see the high degree of deterioration of glucose metabolism *only* because the participants did not eat breakfast [my italics].' But that *wasn't* the only change. In fact, when the patients were skipping breakfast they were on the third day of a weight-loss regime, whereas when they were eating breakfast they were not: unlike Professor Christiansen, Professors Jakubowicz and Froy had not compensated for the breakfasts their patients missed (i.e. they did not increase their food at lunch and dinner) so when they got their patients to skip breakfast they were also putting them on weight-loss diets – reducing their intake from 2,100 to 1,400 calories a day – and measuring the differences only on the third day.

And because the breakfast skippers were losing weight, their blood levels of chemicals called free fatty acids were about twice those of the breakfast eaters.* As we shall see, those are the chemicals that turned their dinners into dangerous meals.

Let's now return to the study that *The Times* reported under the headline 'Diabetics better off with high-energy breakfast'. In that study Professors Jakubowicz and Froy restricted their

---

* It was invaluable of Professors Jakubowicz and Froy to report the levels of free fatty acids but, on a pedantic note, they report them in Fig 1E in pmol/l, and in Table 1 as mmol/l; do they mean μmol/l in both cases?

patients to 1,500 calories a day, and since the reference ranges are around 2,600 calories a day for men, 2,100 for women,[10] and since half the patients in their study were men and half women, they had again put their patients on a weight-loss regime, which would again have raised the circulating levels of free fatty acids, which would again have turned their dinners into dangerous meals, so a more accurate *Times* headline might have been: 'Diabetics *on weight-loss diets* better off with *low-energy dinner* [my italics]'.

To conclude, therefore, *all* blood glucose studies have confirmed that breakfast is a dangerous meal in type 2 diabetics and its associated conditions, but Professors Jakubowicz and Froy have further shown that – under the temporary circumstances of weight-loss dieting – dinner can also become a dangerous meal, perhaps even a very dangerous one. But that is not at all the same thing as saying that breakfast is safe, which – weight-losing or not – it *never* is.

And now that we understand the biochemistry, we can clear up some dietary confusions. So when Professors Daniela Jakubowicz and Oren Froy put ninety-three obese or overweight women with the metabolic syndrome on a three-meals-a-day weight-loss diet (1,400 calories a day) over twelve weeks, the participants lost more weight (8.7 kg vs 3.6 kg) and achieved better blood lipid and insulin-resistance levels if more food was provided at breakfast than at dinner[11] – but that will only have been because their dietary regime had, thanks to the free fatty acids of weight loss, temporarily turned dinner into a dangerous meal.

Equally, when Dr Mauro Lombardo and his colleagues in Rome put thirty-six overweight middle-aged women on a three-meals-and-two-snacks-a-day weight-loss diet (600 calorie daily deficit) he found, as described in the title of his paper, 'Morning meal more efficient for fat loss in a 3-month lifestyle intervention',[12] but that will have been only because Lombardo had also temporarily turned dinner into a dangerous meal. In daily non-weight-loss life, these people would all be much better off skipping breakfast.

Two lessons: There are two lessons to learn from this chapter. First, the most important part of a scientific paper is the 'Methods' section. If you don't examine that carefully, you'll miss the fact that subjects may not just be subjects, they may also be eating fewer calories. But second, don't extrapolate. When the cot death doctors extrapolated from babies in intensive care units to healthy babies, and when the oxygen doctors extrapolated from hypoxic babies to all, they left death and destruction in their wake. Equally, studies on weight-loss regimes should not be extrapolated to normal life, especially as normal life is generally characterised by gentle weight gain.

13

Blood glucose and breakfast: the healthy minority

OK, so blood glucose levels rise dangerously after breakfast in type 2 diabetics and in people who have prediabetes and who are obese; what about in healthy people?

Before answering this question, three well-known pieces of biology need to be rehearsed:

1 High levels of blood glucose are dangerous
2 Insulin is the hormone that lowers blood levels of glucose
3 Yet there are conditions when the body resists the blood glucose lowering effects of insulin. And as we will see, we humans are naturally insulin-resistant in the mornings.

I shall now list the blood glucose breakfast studies in healthy people, below.

The biochemical evidence for breakfast being a dangerous meal in healthy people

- in 1969 Dr Malherbe and his colleagues from the University of Louvain, Belgium, showed that blood levels of insulin in seven healthy subjects were higher after breakfast than after lunch or dinner, even though the blood levels of glucose were similar – i.e. they required more insulin after breakfast to achieve the same degree of glucose control as after lunch and dinner.[1]

In other words, there was resistance to insulin in the morning, meaning that breakfast was a dangerous meal

- in 1988 Dr Kenneth Polonsky and his colleagues from the University of Chicago measured the glucose and insulin responses of fourteen healthy volunteers over a twenty-four-hour period. The volunteers ate three meals a day, with 20 per cent of the calories being consumed at breakfast and with 40 per cent being consumed at lunch and dinner respectively. But, nonetheless, the glucose and insulin responses to all three meals were similar: i.e. breakfast stimulated twice as much of a glucose and insulin response per calorie as did lunch or dinner. Breakfast was therefore a dangerous meal for healthy people: their insulin resistance was higher in the mornings.[2]

- in 2007 Drs Guido Freckmann and Cordelia Haug of the Institute for Diabetes Technology at the University of Ulm, Germany, studied circulating glucose levels in twenty-one young fit adults, and they found that the meal that provoked the highest glucose peak was breakfast, even though its energy content was less than that of the other two meals: i.e. their subjects' insulin resistance was higher in the mornings.[3]

- in a similar study from 2009, Dr Jian Zhou and his colleagues from the Shanghai Diabetes Institute showed that, even when subjects ate only half as many calories at breakfast as at lunch or supper, their peak glucose levels following all three meals were similar.[4] I.e. breakfast was a dangerous meal

- also in 2009, Professor Taylor from Newcastle, UK, broke the overnight fasts of a group of normal subjects in one of two different ways: he either gave them breakfast or he persuaded them not to eat until lunchtime. His subjects' blood glucose and insulin spikes were similar after either meal, but he'd given them 200 fewer calories for breakfast, so clearly there was greater insulin resistance at breakfast time.[5] I.e. breakfast was a dangerous meal

- in yet another 2009 study, Dr Karpe and his colleagues from the Oxford University Centre for Diabetes, on studying blood glucoses over twenty-four hours in eight lean men whose breakfast and lunch carbohydrate contents were the same, found their blood glucose responses were also the same. But 50 per cent more insulin was secreted after breakfast than after lunch, thus showing that insulin resistance was greater at breakfast time than at lunchtime.[6]

The biochemical evidence from these studies is pretty clear: breakfast is a dangerous meal, even for healthy people. But just as it seemed that the story was confirmed, it was challenged. Here are some of the opposing studies:

The biochemical evidence for breakfast being a safe (!) meal in healthy people

- although in 1988 Dr Kenneth Polonsky had found that insulin-resistance was greatest in the morning, in 1992 he reported that if eight normal subjects were asked either to skip lunch, or to eat an additional meal in the middle of the night, their levels of glucose and insulin rose higher in the evenings than the mornings:[7] i.e. following his interventions, Dr Polonky's subjects' evenings became a time of insulin-resistance; i.e. dinner had become a dangerous meal, compared to which breakfast was safer

- in 1999 Dr Linda Morgan of the University of Surrey, UK, on studying nine healthy men whom she had, like Dr Polonsky, asked to skip lunch, also found that their sensitivity to insulin fell during the day, and that in consequence dinner had become a more dangerous meal than breakfast[8]

- and in 2012, on studying the blood glucose and insulin responses of twenty subjects, Dr Ananda Basu and his colleagues from the Mayo College of Medicine, Rochester, found that breakfast emerged as the safest meal of the day. Healthy subjects apparently had a lower insulin-sensitivity in the evening than later in the day, so their blood glucose levels rose over the course of the day.[9]

What's going on? The studies described above seem to be pretty similar in their design, yet they reach very different conclusions. The clue comes from Dr Polonsky's two papers: when in 1988 he'd found breakfast to be a dangerous meal, he'd simply *observed* what happened to people when they ate three conventional meals a day. But when in 1992 he'd found it to be relatively safe, he'd *experimented*: he'd got his subjects to skip lunch, so they were in effect on a weight-loss regime for a day. Since weight loss will raise the blood levels of free fatty acids in the blood, Dr Polonsky had turned his subjects' dinners into dangerous meals.

Which Dr Morgan confirmed. She too got her subjects to skip lunch, so like Dr Polonsky's they too were on a weight-loss regime. Further – and most helpfully – she chronicled the levels of free fatty acids, confirming that they rose markedly over the course of the lunch-free day, and so confirming how she'd turned her subjects' dinner into a dangerous meal.

And in another experiment, Dr Polonsky got his subjects to eat an additional meal in the middle of the night, and we know what happens when you disturb people's sleep: they develop a stressed biochemistry (including rises in free fatty acids)[10], which translates into rises in blood sugar levels.

As for Dr Basu's subjects: well, their average blood glucose levels after lunch were 11.1 mmol/l (and almost as high after dinner and breakfast, 10.8 and 10.3 respectively), and since a person is considered to be diabetic if a random blood glucose level is 11.0 mmol/l (see later), Dr Basu's subjects had apparently become diabetic during his study. Since his study lasted four nights and three days, during which time the subjects were confined to hospital and infused with chemicals through intravenous cannulae while being subjected to six-hour periods of enforced bed rest, the subjects were presumably stressed, which raises insulin-resistance.[11] It is well-known that for a glucose tolerance test: 'You should be normally active, for example not lying down or confined to a bed like a patient in a hospital.'[12]

Aware of this difficulty, Dr Basu got his patients to walk around for some of the day, but with blood glucose levels of 11 we have to assume his regime failed to solve the problem.

To conclude, therefore, simple observation has established that breakfast is a dangerous meal in healthy people, and only by experiments that raise subjects' levels of free fatty acids and/ or stress them have dinners been turned temporarily into even more dangerous meals. But breakfast is *always* a dangerous meal – while dinner becomes so only on weight-losing.

A lesson: This chapter reinforces an old but positive lesson. I've here reinterpreted the findings of a number of scientists, but I've been able to do so only because they reported inconvenient facts (blood glucose levels of 11 mmol/l, abnormal levels of free fatty acids, etc.) so honestly. The only crime in science is dishonesty, and there are no criminals here, only the shifting of paradigms.

14

Why have the scientists claimed breakfast to be safe?

Both the epidemiology and the biochemistry, if interpreted dispassionately, show that breakfast is a dangerous meal, but the interesting question is not 'why is it a dangerous meal?' but, rather, 'why have the scientists apparently misled us?' The epidemiologists have conflated correlation with causation in ways that seem almost perverse, while the biochemists have seemed even worse: in the face of the obvious fact that breakfast is dangerous they have chosen, instead, to distort their subjects' metabolism by finding ways – generally by food restriction – to raise the circulating levels of free fatty acids, thus temporarily turning people's dinners into even more dangerous meals. Having done which, the biochemists have then absolved our daily breakfast instead of damning the weight loser's dinner. Why?

First, let me affirm that the scientists have of course not tried to mislead us, but I do think they have misled themselves. For six reasons: inheritance, common sense, money, virtue-signalling, ownership and collective action.

Inheritance: The medical community inherited the two pro-breakfast mantras and, as Thomas Kuhn argued in his *The Structure of Scientific Revolutions*, scientists dislike shifting paradigms: the old guard dislike acknowledging error, and the new guard – anxious for their grants and publications and promotions – are reluctant to challenge the old guard, so science can too easily adhere to discredited paradigms long after their sell-by dates. Famously, Max Planck wrote in his 1949 *Scientific Autobiography and Other Papers* that 'A new scientific truth does not triumph by convincing its opponents ... but rather because the opponents eventually die' (often paraphrased as 'science advances funeral by funeral').* Or in the words of Professor John Ioannidis of Stanford University, the scholar of science who wrote the 2005 paper 'Why Most Published Research Findings are False': 'for many current scientific fields, claimed research findings may often be simply accurate measures of the existing bias.'[1]

Common sense: In his video explaining why he felt it was his duty to push Americans into eating breakfast, Edward Bernays said, 'the body loses energy during the night and needs it during the day,' which seems to make sense. But in his 1994 book *The Unnatural Nature of Science* the biologist Lewis Wolpert explained how science often flouts common sense – and Bernays's comment is in fact non-sense.

Money: This is self-evident. Huge sums of money are spent by the breakfast companies in sponsoring research papers that rarely tell untruths but which are artful in their selection of data.

Virtue-signalling: Ever since the journalist Albert Shaw wrote in 1891 that to drive the children of the poor to school unfed

---

* Planck's assertion has been confirmed empirically. When a group funded by the National Science Foundation studied the premature deaths of 452 leading scientists, the number of papers published by their collaborators fell precipitously while a significant number of new scientists with new ideas moved into the field, publishing a disproportionate number of novel, much-cited papers (P. Azoulat et al. (2015), 'Does science advance one funeral at a time?', www.econ.upf.edu/~fonsrosen/images/planck_complete_12-02-2015.pdf. Accessed 10 April 2016).

would be like pouring water into a sieve, breakfast has been associated with virtue. Only a bad person would limit social justice, and since everybody 'knows' that governments are always looking to cut budgets, even for free school meals, so – even in the face of inconvenient scientific evidence – good people will support breakfast, particularly as nearly half of all children in America (including 90 per cent of black children) will at some point in their lives be so impoverished as to receive food stamps.[2]

(Actually Parkinson's Law, 'public choice theory' and simple history show that governments are almost always looking to expand their budgets, but – hey – best to be safe.)

Ownership: Because breakfast cereals are widely eaten, and because they are so artificial, nutritionists have adopted them as favoured vehicles by which to supplement the diet of the population. So it has become conventional to enrich and/or fortify (technically, 'enrich' and 'fortify' have different meanings in this context) cereals with a range of vitamins (such as thiamine, niacin, riboflavin and folic acid), minerals (such as iron, zinc and calcium) and other nutrients.

The fortification of foods is not inherently wrong (the iodinisation of table salt has lowered the incidence of goitre; and the fluoridisation of water has reduced the rates of tooth decay), but the idea that products as innately unhealthy as breakfast cereals can be redeemed by their fortification with certain chemicals is unsustainable. We should be encouraging a balanced diet, not pushing unhealthy products that the nutritionists nonetheless feel they 'own' because they've persuaded an agency to supplement them with certain chemicals.

Collective action: Ever since the economist Mancur Olson wrote his *Logic of Collective Action* in 1965, we've known that public opinion is moulded not by the public good but, rather, by special interest groups. The wholesale and retail breakfast caterers have much to gain by shifting public opinion, while the general public has too many other concerns to dedicate time and effort into the investigation of their claims, so by default the only well-funded breakfast lobby is a very interested one indeed.

That lobby is, moreover, only strengthened by government. Ideally, publicly funded scientists would hold industrial researchers to account, but unfortunately governments work to a false paradigm of industrial science needing government support,[3] so instead of seeing their main role as challenging industry, too many government agencies see their role as supporting it. The US federal commitment to industry's welfare was exposed, for example, by Marion Nestle, the professor of nutrition at New York University, when she was hired to edit the 1988 *Surgeon General's Report on Nutrition and Health*: 'My first day on the job, I was given the rules: no matter what the research indicated, the report could not recommend "eat less meat" as a way to reduce the intake of saturated fat, nor could it suggest restrictions on intake of any other category of food.'[4] To this day, as the Harvard University department of nutrition reminds us regularly, too little the federal government says about food or its science can be trusted because it is reluctant to harm the producers.

Nonetheless there have always been credible anti-breakfast voices. From the joint 1973 anti-hypoglycaemia statement of the American Medical and Diabetes Associations and the Endocrine Society, to the individual researchers I cite in this book, there have always been sceptics who have challenged the orthodoxy. Here, I've collated their voices. And I have to collate those voices, because it's not enough to assert that breakfast is a dangerous meal. Without reinterpreting the erroneous conclusions of the past, I'd only be throwing another voice into the maelstrom of opinion, whereas if I show how the work of the past can be reinterpreted and incorporated into a new paradigm, that new paradigm will emerge all the stronger.

Reinterpreting the experiments of others is not a sure-fire way of making friends – and I fear that breakfast scientists and their employers will scour my book for the mistakes I will undoubtedly have made – but because we scientists are, contrary to myth, verifiers rather than falsifiers,* there seems to be no other way for the enterprise to advance.

---

* People believe that Karl Popper's *Logic of Scientific Discovery* describes a world in which researchers love to have their work disproved or in which they love to disprove that of others. Far from it. Researchers hate having their own work disproved, and they don't like to make enemies either.

PART SEVEN

How Breakfast Kills Us

Breakfast kills us because the
authorities have been misleading
us for over half a century.

15

The fat saga

The modern dietary era was launched in 1953 when Ancel Keys published his crucial paper suggesting that fat in the diet precipitated atherosclerosis.[1]

America, post-war, was engulfed by a wave of fatal heart attacks and strokes, to which everyone seemed vulnerable (F.D. Roosevelt had died in 1945 at the age of 63 from a stroke), and the nation was looking for solutions. So in 1948 President Truman helped launch the famous Framingham Heart Study (which, three generations and 1,200 papers later, is still running), trusting that an analysis of the lifestyles of the population of the small Massachusetts town of Framingham might help reveal the causes of heart attacks and strokes. But in 1953 Keys pre-empted its findings by arguing that, because atherosclerotic plaques were cholesterol-rich, they might be caused by fatty food.

Ancel Keys (1904–2004) was a man to whom, unfortunately, people listened. A professor at the University of Minnesota, he made his first memorable advance in 1942 when he developed K-rations (the K is said to be for Keys, though that might be a myth) to provide soldiers on active service with 3,200 calories daily in a pack that weighed only 28 oz (790 g). He went on to perform his famous Minnesota Starvation Experiment (discussed above) to help understand how to treat the millions of starving people the war generated.

His fat theory, moreover, made sense (thus reminding us that H.L. Mencken said that for every complex problem there is a solution that is clear, simple and wrong). The two key dietary fats, Keys suggested, were cholesterol and triglyceride. His model of

dietary cholesterol → circulating cholesterol → atherosclerosis

seemed obvious, but his other model of

dietary triglyceride → circulating cholesterol → atherosclerosis

seemed not so obvious, yet it appeared that dietary triglyceride in some way stimulated the body to synthesise more cholesterol.

By 1955, though, Keys and others had appreciated that dietary cholesterol is not a human danger: our livers synthesise most of our cholesterol, and when we ingest it in our food our livers simply turn down their synthetic rate.[2] That negative feedback is not true of all animals, particularly not of herbivores such as rabbits, which – because plants are low in cholesterol – do not normally handle significant amounts of it. So herbivores, when fed high cholesterol in the laboratory, respond with raised cholesterol in the blood: their livers don't know any better. But we are omnivores, our livers are not naive, and when fed high cholesterol we do not respond with raised levels of blood cholesterol. So for us:

dietary cholesterol ≠ circulating cholesterol

Keys, though, never retracted his suggestion that dietary triglycerides stimulate cholesterol synthesis, and this remains the official position. Keys proposed the relationship because, when he graphed the total fat content in the diet of six different countries, ranging from Japan (7 per cent fat in the diet) through to the USA (40 per cent) the death rates from heart disease of 55–59-year-olds rose accordingly, from 0.5 per thousand in Japan to just under 7 per thousand in the USA.

There was just one problem with that graph. In 1965 Ronald Reagan published an autobiography entitled *Where's the Rest of Me?* after his famous line in the 1942 film *Kings Row*. Well, where was the rest of Keys's data?

Keys's figures came from published international data sets, but he had selected only six countries. Why? Shockingly (no other adverb will do), to give the result he wanted. So when in 1957 a British physiologist called John Yudkin extended the study to encompass the rest of the available data, on twenty-two countries, he found that from:

> all the information available from international statistics [there is only] a moderate but by no means excellent relationship between fat consumption and coronary mortality . . . A better relationship turned out to exist between sugar consumption and coronary mortality in a variety of countries. The best relationship of all existed between the number of reported coronary deaths in the UK and the rise in the number of radio and television sets.[3]

The last, apparently mischievous, observation has been confirmed. Pooling all the published data, a Danish/Harvard group showed recently that every two hours spent watching television a day increases the chances of developing:

- type 2 diabetes by 20 per cent
- cardiovascular disease by 15 per cent
- dying from any cause by 13 per cent.[4]

Although we cannot exclude the idea that unhealthy people may preferentially watch TV, the causative link presumably goes:

watch TV ➔ neglect exercise and/ ➔ become unhealthy*
                or snack too much

---

* Presumably by acquiring the metabolic syndrome; see later.

In his attack on sugar and defence of fats (he wrote of 'good nutritious foods like meat and cheese and milk')[5] Yudkin was not quite alone. Supporting him were Drs Jacob Yerushalmy and Herman Hilleboe, from Berkeley and the New York State Commission of Health, who also complained that Keys had selected his data.[6] Meanwhile Drs Pete Ahrens of Rockefeller University, New York, and Margaret Albrink, of Yale University, found a stronger correlation between raised blood levels of *triglycerides* and heart disease than between raised cholesterol and heart disease. *And* they found that carbohydrate in the diet raised triglyceride levels. So their model was:

| dietary carbohydrates | → | converted by the liver into blood triglycerides | → | heart disease[7] |

Meanwhile Dr George Mann of Vanderbilt University found during the 1960s that the Masai people in Kenya ate little but fatty meat, and drank little but full-fat milk, yet had almost no cardiovascular disease and had startlingly low circulating blood cholesterol levels. So his model was:

fat in the diet → no problem[8]

Stung by these critics, Keys responded not by reasoned argument but with abuse, writing in the journal *Atherosclerosis* that the sugar idea was a 'mountain of nonsense'.[9] Nonetheless he embarked on his famous *Seven Countries Study*, which he published in 1970, where he personally determined what people were eating in Italy, Greece, Yugoslavia, Finland, the Netherlands, Japan and the USA. He refined his surveys to look at saturated (i.e. animal) fats rather than total fats, and yet again he found a strong association between (saturated) fat ingestion and deaths from heart disease.[10]

But when one of his colleagues, Alessandro Menotti, re-analysed the data after twenty-five years' further study, he found that 'sweets' (sugar-rich products, cakes and other confectioneries) in the diet correlated more strongly with coronary mortality than did 'animal food' (butter, meat, eggs, margarine, lard, milk and cheese), thus indicating that even Keys's own programme of work suggested that it was carbohydrates, not fats, that killed people.[11]

Keys had cheated, and the best exposure of his malfeasances was provided by Nina Teicholz in her recent book *The Big Fat Surprise* where she also chronicled how, during the 1960s, a series of epidemiological studies failed to confirm the fat hypothesis.[12] Meanwhile in 1972 John Yudkin published his brilliant book *Pure, White and Deadly* (which refers of course to sugar).

Yet Keys won the argument, not because of his venom, nor even because of his own science, but because of a tide in other researchers' science. Dr Robert Lustig of the University of California, San Francisco, is the author of the 2013 anti-sugar book *Fat Chance: Beating the Odds against Sugar, Processed Food, Obesity and Disease*, and here is an extract from his introduction to the 2012 reissue of Yudkin's *Pure, White and Deadly*:

> Three scientific findings of the 1970s undid Yudkin's case and sealed his fate. Firstly, by studying the genetic disease familial hypercholesterolaemia (victims experience heart attacks as early as eighteen years old), Michael Brown and Joseph Goldstein discovered low-density lipoproteins (LDL) and the LDL receptor (which won them the Nobel Prize), leading to the hypothesis that LDL was the bad actor in heart disease. Secondly, dietary studies showed that dietary fat raised LDL levels. Thirdly, large epidemiological studies showed that LDL levels correlate with heart disease in populations. Slam dunk, right? It's the fat, stupid.
>
> . . . But . . . there wasn't one type of LDL, there were two: large buoyant LDL, driven by dietary fat, but which was neutral in terms of heart disease; and small dense LDL, driven by dietary carbohydrate, and which oxidises quickly, driving atherosclerotic plaque formation.[13]

That is to say cholesterol is transported by LDLs in the blood, but the large LDLs (which are raised by saturated fat) are apparently neutral in terms of heart disease: our killers are the small LDL subtypes of the metabolic syndrome (see later).

The role of government: Keys's errors were, unfortunately, reinforced by government. In 1977 the US Senate Select Committee on Nutrition and Human Needs published its *Dietary Goals for the United States*, which represented the federal government's first official advice on diet. In the words of the committee's chairman, Senator George McGovern: 'We as a government . . . have an obligation to provide practical guides to the individual consumer as well as set national dietary goals for the country.'

The committee's *Goals* included:

1 Increase carbohydrate consumption to account for 55 to 60 per cent of the energy (caloric) intake
2 Reduce overall fat consumption from approximately 40 to 30 per cent energy intake
3 Reduce saturated fat consumption to account for about 10 per cent of total energy intake
4 Reduce cholesterol consumption to about 300 mg a day.*

And in 1983 the British government followed suit by publishing similar advice. Yet there was, even then, considerable doubt about the fat hypothesis, and in 1977 the American Medical Association responded to the *Goals* with: 'The evidence for assuming that benefits to be derived from the adoption of such universal dietary goals . . . is not conclusive, and there is potential for harmful effects.'[14]

Moreover, a recent study has confirmed that when the US

---

* Depressingly, we now know that the Harvard scientists who advised the Senate Committee received secret fees from the sugar industry (C.E. Kearns et al. (12 September 2016), 'Sugar industry and coronary heart disease: A historical analysis of internal industry documents', *JAMA Intern Med*, doi:10.1001/jamainternmed.2016.5394.)

federal and British governments introduced their low-fat, high-carbohydrate dietary guidelines, the best evidence then available did *not* support the idea that a low-fat diet was good for people; that idea was always an unwarranted extrapolation from Ancel Keys.[15]

The only responsible reaction to the scientific uncertainty would have been a confession of ignorance; instead of which the Senate committee acknowledged ignorance, but – on invoking the example of Marc Lalonde MP – it still determined on giving advice:

> Marc Lalonde, Canada's Minister of National Health and Welfare, said: 'Even such a simple question as whether one should severely limit his consumption of butter and eggs can be a matter of endless scientific debate . . . [so] it would be easy for health educators and promoters to sit on their hands . . . But many of Canada's health problems are sufficiently pressing that action has to be taken even if all the scientific evidence is not in.'

In 1974 Lalonde had indeed published a working paper entitled *A New Perspective on the Health of Canadians* which was, in effect, a manifesto justifying the intrusion of the federal government in Ottawa into the lifestyles and diets of Canadians, but the statement that 'action has to be taken even if all the scientific evidence is not in' is the very definition of irresponsibility. All science is of course only provisional, but to issue official advice knowing that debate is still raging is to invert the very nature of science: it is to cherry-pick a conclusion that is not backed by the research, which can lead to conclusions that are 100 per cent wrong. As in this case it did.

Correcting Keys: It was Atkins and his diet that rescued humanity from Keys's errors. Dr Robert Atkins (1930–2003) was the New York cardiologist who, troubled by his own obesity, had read a paper in the *Journal of the American Medical Association* that recommended that slimmers should ditch carbohydrates for meat.[16] He tried it, it worked for him, and in 1972 he published *Dr Atkins' Diet Revolution* which advocated the eating of meat, eggs, cream and milk. This was a revolution indeed,* yet it seemed to work better for weight loss than did conventional low-fat diets.[17] And it also seemed to be better for people's health.

Thus did Atkins launch today's insurgency; and the evidence for dietary carbohydrate, not fat, being our major killer, is growing. I've collated the findings of a series of recent papers below.

———————

Fat versus carbohydrate as the major cardiac killer: some recent studies

- the celebrated Spanish PREDIMED study on 7,447 subjects aged 55–88, who between them collected a total of 288 heart attacks or strokes over 4.8 years, showed that high-fat Mediterranean diets lower the chances of a cardiovascular event by 30 per cent compared with conventional low-fat (i.e. high-carbohydrate) diets[18]

- a Portuguese/US collaboration reviewing the findings on a total of 1,141 obese patients, who had been studied by seventeen different groups, found that on low-carbohydrate (i.e. high-fat) diets, they dramatically improved their:
  - weights, BMIs and waist circumferences
  - blood pressures

———————

* Though as early as 1867, in his *Letter on Corpulence Addressed to the Public*, William Banting, a London undertaker who was apparently a distant ancestor of Frederick Banting of insulin fame, had advocated a low-carbohydrate diet for weight loss. Gary Taubes opened his excellent 2007 book *Good Calories, Bad Calories* with the William Banting story, which can also be found at http://second-opinions.ginwiz.com/Ink000/=www.second-opinions.co.uk/banting.html/.

     – blood glucose, insulin and HbA1c levels
     – plasma triglyceride and HDL levels
     – inflammatory markers.[19]

- a German group found that when forty type 2 diabetics were placed on low-carbohydrate diets, they achieved 'remarkable'* drops in their HbA1cs[20]

- a US group found that when patients with the metabolic syndrome were put on high-fat low-carbohydrate weight-loss diets, their:
     – insulin levels fell by half and insulin sensitivity rose by half
     – glucose levels and weight moved dramatically into healthier ranges
     – triglyceride levels fell by 50 per cent
     – HDL levels rose by 50 per cent
     – inflammatory markers, too, fell further on the high-fat rather than the low-fat diet.[21]

- an international group found that, even on full-calorie diets, patients with the metabolic syndrome do better on low-carbohydrate food[22]

- when the famous 2007 'A TO Z' Stanford study compared the effects of four diets:
     – Atkins (35 per cent carbohydrate)
     – Zone (46 per cent carbohydrate)
     – LEARN** (47 per cent carbohydrate)
     – Ornish (52 per cent carbohydrate)

---

* Since 1980 scientists' language has become more dramatic, and words such as 'remarkable' are now used eight times more in research papers than thirty-five years ago (C.H. Vinkers et al., 2015, 'Use of positive and negative words in scientific PubMed abstracts between 1974 and 2014: retrospective analysis', *BMJ* 351:h6467). And why not?
** LEARN was a *t*raditional diet, hence the T in 'A TO Z'.

it found that the lower the carbohydrate in the diet, the lower
were:
   – the blood triglycerides
   – glucose
   – insulin
   – weight
   – blood pressure
   – and the higher was the HDL cholesterol.[23]
The study also showed that the higher-fat lower-carbohydrate
diets raised the blood LDL-cholesterol, but only of the large
LDL particles, which are relatively safe

- epidemiological surveys, moreover, confirm the dangers of
  carbohydrates. Consider rice. Emily Hu and her colleagues
  from Harvard found, on pooling the global data, that 'Each
  serving per day of white rice consumption was associated with
  an 11% increase in risk of diabetes.'[24] So although the obesity
  rate in Japan, at 3 per cent, is only a tenth of the USA's, and
  although the average Japanese citizen consumes 200 calories
  a day less than the average American, and although the level
  of physical activity in Japan is significantly higher than in
  America (the Japanese use public transport more than do
  Americans, which involves more walking)[25] the Japanese rate
  of type 2 diabetes is disproportionately high at 7.3 per cent,[26]
  which seems to be attributable to the high rate of consumption
  of rice.[27]

Official dietary advice today: Despite the recent research, the
official advice remains pro-carbohydrate and anti-fat. Here are
the current NHS recommendations for healthy people:

Base your meals on starchy food. Starchy foods should
make up about one third of the foods you eat. Starchy
foods include potatoes, cereals, pasta, rice and bread . . .

> Most of us should eat more starchy foods: try to include at
> least one starchy food with each main meal. Some people
> think starchy foods are fattening, but gram for gram the
> carbohydrate they contain provides fewer than half the
> calories of fat.[28]

That is not a rogue NHS web page. Another page recommends that 'starchy foods such as potatoes, bread, cereals, rice and pasta should make up about a third of the food you eat.'[29]

Healthy Americans are urged to eat even more carbohydrates, and the *2010–2015 Dietary Guidelines for Americans*[30] produced jointly by the US Department of Agriculture and the US Department of Health and Human Services recommends that all Americans, from the age of 1 onwards, should consume between 45 and 65 per cent of their food as carbohydrates (for the *2015–2020 Guidelines* see p. 121).

If healthy people are to eat carbohydrates, what are type 2 diabetics to eat? The same! In the past, type 2s were urged to avoid sugar and carbohydrates, and instead to eat special 'diabetic' (i.e. low-sugar) foods, but that advice has since been superseded. In the words of Diabetes UK:

> 'Diabetic' foods became popular in the 1960s when diabetes
> care focused on eating a sugar-free diet. Since the 1980s,
> dietary recommendations have moved away from a sugar-free
> diet . . . but the myth that people with diabetes shouldn't eat
> sugar still persists. The truth is that people with diabetes can
> consume sugar . . . The guidelines also advise against the use
> of 'diabetic' foods.[31]

In the words of the American Diabetic Association:

> MYTH: People with diabetes need to follow a special diet.
> FACT: People with diabetes benefit from the same healthy diet
> that is good for everyone else . . . with a limited amount of
> fat.[32]

So diabetics are now advised to eat similar food, including carbohydrates, as healthy people. Here is Diabetes UK's *Eating Well With Type 2 Diabetes*:

> **At each meal include starchy carbohydrate foods** such as bread, pasta, chapatis, potatoes, yam, noodles, rice and cereals . . . Eating sugar doesn't cause diabetes and people with diabetes do not need a sugar-free diet . . . All breakfast cereals are fine. More filling choices, like porridge and All-Bran or fruit and fibre will see you through the morning. Add semi-skimmed or skimmed milk . . . fruit juice can count towards one of your five a day . . . Bread, toast, bread muffins and crumpets are good alternatives to cereal . . . Ordinary jams and marmalades . . . are okay too [bold type in the original].

Equally, the American Diabetes Association recommends that patients with type 2 diabetes should eat 'about 45–60 grams of carbohydrate at a meal [i.e. approximately a third of their calorie intake]'.[33]

This emphasis on carbohydrates, of course, is inspired by the belief that we should reduce our intake of the other major calorie-rich food, namely fat, so Diabetes UK advises: '**Cut down on the fat you eat,** particularly saturated fats, as a low fat diet benefits health . . . As fat is the greatest source of calories, eating less will help you to lose weight [bold type in the original].' And as we saw above, the American Diabetes Association offers similar advice ('with a limited amount of fat').

This pro-carbohydrate advice *must* be wrong. Type 2 diabetics should obviously avoid carbohydrates because the disease is one of glucose intolerance, yet even healthy people should surely avoid them: their consumption will raise blood glucose levels, and there is no such thing as a safe raised level of blood glucose, even within the normal range. So a survey of middle-aged men in Norfolk, UK, found that the best predictor of their deaths from cardiovascular disease wasn't their level of cholesterol, weight or blood pressure, it was their blood glucose levels, measured as something called HbA1c (see p.121) – and the correlation applied even within the normal range (i.e. high normal blood glucose levels are dangerous).[34] There appears to be no such thing as a safe blood glucose molecule.

Pre-Keys, the authorities were rational. The greatest physician of his age was Sir William Osler (1849–1919) of successively McGill University, Johns Hopkins Hospital and Oxford University, and his *Principles and Practice of Medicine*, first published in 1892, was for forty years the leading textbook because it adopted the unusual approach of advocating treatments based on scientific observation rather than on myth and custom. In consequence, it recommended relatively few treatments, but one treatment it did recommend was that diabetics' diet should not exceed 5 per cent carbohydrate.[35]

More on the official dietary advice

Sometimes I almost feel sorry for the official bodies, because they remain wedded to their pro-carbohydrate anti-fat narrative, yet they cannot ignore the latest science. So although the *2015–2020 Dietary Guidelines for Americans* did not dramatically change the recommendations of the *2010–2015 Guidelines* (continuing to advise that 'healthy eating patterns include . . . starchy and other vegetables'), the *2015–2020 Guidelines* nonetheless recognise sugar and refined carbohydrates as problematic. Even so, when they recommend we consume less than 10 per cent of calories daily from added sugar, we need to ask why that figure isn't 0 per cent, and when they recommend that at least half the grains we eat should be whole grains, we should actually be sceptical about all grains. And in continuing to recommend we eat fat-free dairy products (which are supplemented with sugar) and to consume fruit juices (whose sugar may be unleavened by fibre) and to limit our consumption of trans fats (their consumption should be zero) the *2015–2020 Guidelines* remain in many respects positively unhelpful.[36]

It was also unhelpful to read in the *New York Times* for 18 January 2016 that the early drafts of the *2015–2020 Guidelines* confirmed that red and processed meats increase the risks of developing bowel and other cancers but that – following the lobbying of Congress by the National Cattlemen's Beef Association – this reference was removed from the final version.[37] Moreover, where the *Guidelines* recommend that less than 10 per cent of daily calories should come from saturated or animal fats, we should remember that these increasingly appear to be cardiac neutral rather than dangerous: and if they are to be replaced, they should be replaced with unsaturated plant fats, which seem to be positively healthy, and not with carbohydrate.[38] Nuts not fries.

Nor need we fret for those spurned carbohydrates: as the nutritionist Dr Sarah Schenker told *The Times* on 19 March 2016, if we avoid all sugars and carbohydrates, we're 'not going to get withdrawal symptoms. There'll be no headaches or sweats and your body produces its own sugar . . . so it's not going to have any detrimental effects.'

It was also odd that it was not until 2015 that the US federal government's Dietary Guidelines Advisory Committee reversed its long-standing condemnation of high-cholesterol foods such as eggs, shrimps and lobster, and passed them as safe for human consumption.[39] It took the DGAC so long to recognise what the scientific community (but not unfortunately the general public) had recognised decades ago because proving a negative is so difficult, but perhaps the DGAC shouldn't try to prove negatives: the DGAC might have done the public more good by simply noting that the original dietary cholesterol claim lacked proper scientific support.

There is now such concern over the *Guidelines'* advice on carbohydrates and fat that in 2015 Congress, citing concerns over 'the scientific integrity of the process', and asking for 'full transparency, a lack of bias, and the inclusion of all the latest available research . . . even that which challenges current dietary recommendations', commissioned the National Academy of Medicine (at a cost of $1 million) to review 'the entire process used' to generate the *Guidelines*.[40]

Of the carbohydrates, sugar seems the most dangerous. So the Nurses' Health Studies found that the 'higher consumption of sugar-sweetened beverages is associated with a greater magnitude of weight gain and an increased risk [nearly double] for development of type 2 diabetes.'[41]

Meanwhile a similar European study found that the daily consumption of one can of a commercially sweetened drink increased the risk of developing type 2 diabetes by 18 per cent.[42] Equally, Robert Lustig found that, whereas an increase of 150 calories in a person's diet was associated with a rise of only 0.1 per cent in diabetes, an increase by one can of fizzy drinks a day (which also delivers 150 calories, but in the form of sugar) was associated with a 1.1 per cent increase in diabetes prevalence, which was significant.[43]

Nonetheless, for all the indications of sugar and the carbohydrates as dangerous, the bulk of the evidence points more to their partner in crime – insulin – being the mass killer of western societies. In particular, the condition of 'insulin-resistance' seems to be the major culprit. And since the dangers of breakfast are in large part mediated by insulin, so the two debates of fat/carbohydrate and of breakfast skipping/not skipping find themselves intertwined, which is why the next chapter reports on the carbohydratisation of the English-speaking breakfast.

Cuba

People have questioned the dangers of sugar by pointing to Cuba, and in his superb 2015 book *The Diet Myth* Professor Tim Spector of King's College London wrote: 'Cubans, despite eating on average twice the total amount of sugar as Americans, are poorer but far healthier.'[44]

But a study on sugar uptake over 173 countries, performed by scientists from the universities of California, London, Cambridge and Copenhagen, concluded that 'high sugar producers such as

Brazil, Jamaica, Dominica, Costa Rica, Cuba, Mexico, Trinidad and Tobago . . . experience some of the highest rates of diabetes.'[45]

Fascinatingly, Cuba recently became healthier, not because of its sugar but because of its new-found poverty. The collapse of the Soviet Union robbed it of its largest trading partner, and after 1989 its per capita daily food intake fell from 2,899 to 1,868 calories, while the loss of oil imports forced people away from the internal combustion engine and onto their feet or bicycles, so the proportion of physically active adults rose from 30 to 67 per cent. And the consequence was that the death rates from:

- diabetes fell by 51 per cent
- coronary heart disease by 35 per cent
- stroke by 20 per cent.[46]

Meanwhile the rate of obesity fell from 14 to 7 per cent, and the average BMI fell by 1.5. The lessons are obvious: Cubans are currently healthy *despite* their high sugar consumption, because their consumption of everything else is so modest and because they are forced to exercise. But Cubans are rapidly becoming less healthy again: a series of sad papers in the Cuban medical journal *MEDICC Review* reveals that as the islanders increasingly revert to their traditional, unhealthy meat- and fast-food-based diet, so the current 60 per cent of deaths that are attributable to heart disease, cancer and cerebrovascular diseases is set to rise.[47] As the saying goes, 'Cubans live like the poor but die like the rich' from the heart attacks, strokes and cancer that constitute the disease profile of the west.

The evidence is growing, therefore, that a healthy diet is a low-carbohydrate diet. And dissenting voices that advocate low-carbohydrate (and therefore high-fat) diets are arising even within the 'official' community. In a remarkable 2014 book, *Reverse Your Diabetes*, Dr David Cavan urges type 2 diabetics (and all of us actually) to eschew carbohydrates.[48] Yet Dr Cavan works for the International Diabetes Federation (IDF) – and the IDF is the worldwide alliance of over 230 national diabetes associations including the American Diabetes Association and Diabetes UK, which are among carbohydrate's biggest official supporters. This tolerance speaks well of the scientific openness of the international diabetic community. (Dr Cavan's book, incidentally, is the best book I can recommend for newly diagnosed type 2 diabetics. And, no, I do not know Dr Cavan.)*

Envoi: Nina Teicholz wrote that if there is a Great Man theory of history then 'in the history of nutrition Ancel Keys was by far the Greatest Man,'[49] and on 13 January 1961 he even appeared on the front page of *Time* magazine, which then represented the apogee of American celebrity (though Nixon appeared there fifty-five times, and Hitler was *Time*'s person of the year in 1938, as was Stalin twice, in 1939 and 1942, so *Time*'s take on celebrity is no guarantee of virtue or wisdom or of scientific integrity).

Keys eventually retired to southern Italy where, consuming a Mediterranean diet rich in olive oil, he lived to be just two months short of 101.** But his legacy to the world was not just the demonisation of fat in the diet, but – because people have to eat *something*, and because there's a limit to how much meat they'll eat – also the carbohydratisation of western food, including breakfast. Which has been a disaster.

Ancel Keys not only got his epidemiology wrong, he also got his history and literature wrong. Had he been a classicist he might have known of the ancient Greeks' wise suspicion of

---

* But Dr Cavan is not perfect, and he supposes breakfast to be a healthy meal. Indeed he eats Greek yoghurt, which contains sugar, for breakfast.

** A Mediterranean diet is rich in olive oil, vegetables, fruit, nuts and legumes (peas, beans, lentils, chickpeas); moderate in fish, poultry, alcohol and wholegrain cereals; and low in red meat, processed meat and sweet foods such as cakes or jams.

sugar. In paragraph 404b of Plato's *Republic*, Socrates says that: 'At their feasts Homer feeds his heroes on roast meat, but he never mentions sweet desserts or sweet sauces. In proscribing them, though, he is not unusual, because all professional athletes know that for a man to be in good condition . . . Athenian confectionery is to be avoided.'

Had Keys been an English major, he might have learned of the long English suspicion of sugar. In *Henry IV, Part 1*, Shakespeare has Prince Henry attack Falstaff for being an:

old fat man; a tun of man is thy companion. Why
dost thou converse with that trunk of humours, that
bolting-hutch of beastliness, that swollen parcel
of dropsies, that huge bombard of sack [sweet wine], that stuffed
cloak-bag of guts, that roasted Manningtree ox with
the pudding in his belly

(Act 2, scene 4)

To which Falstaff, that preternatural biochemist, replies:

If sack and sugar be a fault,
God help the wicked!

Dr David Ludwig

Dr David Ludwig of the Children's Hospital, Boston, is an anti-carbohydrate hero. Consider 'adaptive thermogenesis', which – as I reported earlier – is a menace because it encourages weight gain after dieting. Yet in 2012 Dr Ludwig showed that a low-carbohydrate diet – by reversing insulin-resistance – also reverses adaptive thermogenesis.[50]

In his study Dr Ludwig warned that an extremely low carbohydrate diet could raise circulating blood levels of cortisol and the pro-inflammatory compound CRP (C-reactive protein), but he couldn't have been particularly worried because on 29 November 2015 he published an article in the *New York Times* urging the Department of Agriculture in its forthcoming *Dietary Guidelines for Americans 2015–2020* to 'jettison the traditional emphasis on low-fat [i.e. high-carbohydrate] diets'. Unfortunately the USDA ignored him.

Dr Ludwig has also shown that the people who respond best to a low-carbohydrate diet are those with the greatest degree of insulin-resistance; but for reasons that are not fully understood, not all overweight or obese people are insulin-resistant (see later), and a Colorado group has shown that non-insulin-resistant people lose weight better on traditional low-fat diets.[51] To get the best results, therefore, we should perhaps separate people into insulin-resistant and non-insulin-resistant, and provide them with personalised diets.

Personalisation is the future: long-standing vegetarian populations in countries such as India, for example, have evolved different forms of fat metabolism from people from Inuit and Caucasian populations,[52] so diets that are good for some populations may be bad for others: let us admit that there is much we still do not know and let us not rush to over-firm prescriptions. Ancel Keys is in his grave; let's keep his dogmatism there.

———————————

PART EIGHT

Insulin, the Great Traitor

Insulin is an essential hormone,
and without it we die. But in excess
it turns on us and kills us. Breakfast,
sadly, is a source of that excess.

16

The carbohydratisation of the English-speaking breakfast

Breakfast has carbohydratised. After decades of official fat-demonisation, our breakfasts have been carbohydratised and thus turned into weapons of mass insulinisation.

A study from the department of nutrition, University of North Carolina, Chapel Hill, has chronicled the changes in breakfast in the USA over the years 1965–91. The subjects were adults over the age of 18.

TABLE 16.1
Grams of food consumed at breakfast. US adults

Year	1965	1991
Whole milk	105.8	44.1
Low-fat milk	6.9	73.0
Eggs	26.0	12.3
Bacon	4.1	1.1
Bread	30.7	22.0
Ready-to-eat cereals	7.0	14.4
Fruit	48.9	59.4
Fruit juices	7.5	8.6
Butter	3.1	0.7
Margarine	2.4	1.9

Data from P. Haines et al. (1996), 'Trends in breakfast consumption of US adults between 1965–1991', *J Am Diet Assoc* 96: 464–70. The surveys were performed by asking 6,274 people in 1965, and 10,812 in 1989/1991 (and 18,033 in 1977/1978) what they ate for breakfast.

The trends over twenty-five years are obvious. The consumption of animal protein-rich foods (bacon and eggs) more than halved from 30.1 to 13.4 g, the consumption of fat-rich foods (whole milk/butter/margarine) followed a similar trend, while the consumption of ready-to-eat cereals doubled. The consumption of fruit and juices also rose. Not reported was the consumption of sugar, but if the consumption of ready-to-eat cereals doubled, we can suppose that its consumption will also have risen, which presumably will have compensated, carbohydrate-wise (and certainly glycaemic-wise) for the fall in bread consumption. Breakfast has been carbohydratised.

A similar study has been performed by the same department of nutrition on children and adolescents under the age of 18, and Table 16.2 highlights the big changes over time.

TABLE 16.2
Grams of food consumed at breakfast. US children

Year	1965	1991
High-fat milk	181.6	79.5
Low-fat milk	9.1	99.4
Eggs	20.8	11.5
Bacon	3.2	0.96
Bread	29.8	22.1
Pasta/rice/cooked cereals	22.0	21.5
Ready-to-eat cereals	10.3	19.5
Fruit	48.0	55.0
Juices	7.5	15.5
Butter	2.8	0.4
Margarine	2.5	1.6
Cheese	0.7	1.8

Data from A.M. Siega-Riz et al. (1998), 'Trends in breakfast consumption for children in the United States from 1965–1991', *Am J Clin Nutr 67* (suppl): 748S–56S. The surveys were performed by asking 7,513 people in 1965, and 4,289 in 1989/1991 (and 12,561 in 1977/1978) what they ate for breakfast.

The trends over twenty-five years for under-18s are similar to those for over-18s. The consumption of animal protein-rich foods (bacon and eggs) halved from 24 to 12.5 g, the consumption of fat-rich foods (high-fat milk/butter/margarine and cheese) followed a similar trend, while the consumption of ready-to-eat cereals and of fruit and juices nearly doubled. Not reported was the consumption of sugar (the research was supported by the Kellogg company), but if the consumption of ready-to-eat cereals nearly doubled (as did the consumption of juices) then – as above – we can see that its consumption will also have risen, which presumably will have compensated, carbohydrate-wise (and certainly glycaemic-wise) for the fall in bread consumption.

That breakfast has been carbohydratised was confirmed by a 1997 review of a large number of epidemiological studies, which found that 'breakfast consumption . . . is associated with lower intakes of fat and higher intakes of carbohydrate.'[1] Ironically, that was written in praise of breakfast, because people then supposed that fat was dangerous and carbohydrates were benign. But now that we're shifting the paradigm back to the pre-Keys era of Yudkin's 'good nutritious foods like meat and cheese and milk' we reinterpret those data differently. Yet the data are still good.

Breakfast thus straddles both of today's paradigm shifts of carbohydrate/fat and of breakfast skipping/not skipping, and we are recognising it to be not only dangerous in its own right but also because of its content. As an American friend said to me recently, 'The modern American breakfast, with its waffles and cereals and toast and jams, is dessert.' To understand, therefore, why breakfast is doubly dangerous, we need to understand not only why eating in the mornings is dangerous but also why carbohydrates are dangerous.

The two dangers are linked by a common mechanism: insulin.

17

Nothing about breakfast makes sense except in the light of insulin

In a famous phrase Theodosius Dobzhansky said in 1973 that 'Nothing in biology makes sense except in the light of evolution.' Equally, nothing about breakfast – and its dangers – makes sense except in the light of insulin. If we are to understand why breakfast is a dangerous meal, therefore, we have to understand insulin, and our best introduction to it comes from diabetes mellitus.

Diabetes mellitus: Diabetes is an old disease. During the second century AD (CE) Aretaeus of Cappadocia wrote a clinical description that will be recognised by any doctor, nurse or patient today: 'Diabetes . . . is a melting down of the flesh and limbs into urine. The patients never stop making water and the flow is incessant, like the opening of aqueducts. Life is short, unpleasant and painful. The patients' thirst is unquenchable, their drinking is excessive . . . and within a short time they expire.'[1]

He went on to write that 'The disease appears to have got its name from the Greek for siphon.' That was because, Aretaeus explained, the disease is characterised by diuresis or excessive peeing; the words 'diuresis' or 'diuretic' derive from the Greek words for 'through' and 'urine'.

Following the fall of the Roman Empire and the descent of

Europe into the Dark Ages (the early medieval period) scholarship was aborted, and no further advances on Aretaeus's clinical description of diabetes were made until the seventeenth century, when Dr Thomas Willis (1621–75) of Oxford started the process by which the disease was classified into two major categories, diabetes insipidus and diabetes mellitus.*

Diabetes insipidus does not concern us here. Because in Arataeus's day a disease was called 'diabetes' if it involved a diuresis or an excess of urine, diabetes inspidus retains the name but it's fundamentally different from the disease that does concern us, namely mellitus. The obvious distinction is that in mellitus the urine is sweet (because it's full of glucose; 'mellitus' coming from the Greek *meli* for 'honey') whereas in insipidus it's, well, insipid, and not sweet. In the past the differential diagnosis was made by doctors tasting the urine, the task generally being delegated to the most junior member of the team. Insipidus is caused by failures in the antidiuretic hormone system, and it bears no relation to mellitus except that both, for different reasons, produce a diuresis. We'll say no more about diabetes insipidus.

The next major advance in the understanding of diabetes mellitus came in 1889. The pancreas (or sweetbread) is an organ that nestles towards the back of the abdomen (the word 'pancreas' is a Latin adaptation of the Greek for 'all flesh') and in 1889 Oskar Minkowski and Joseph von Mering, in Strasbourg,

---

* Interestingly, although academic science and the liberal arts were extinguished by the fall of the Roman Empire, technology accelerated. The so-called Dark Ages were not dark when it came to developing the crank, the plough, windmills, the harnessing of horses and other techniques of industrial and agricultural progress. The Roman Empire, like the Hellenistic age that preceded it, may have been culturally rich, but it was a slave society that in consequence was technologically stagnant, and we can root our current prosperities in the technologies that emerged, unsung by intellectuals and independent of academic science, during the early medieval period. See my book *Sex, Science and Profits* (2008), William Heinemann, London.

wondered what would happen to a dog if they removed it. What happened was that, among other problems, the dog developed the thirst, peeing and weight loss of diabetes mellitus.[2] The disease seemed to be located, therefore, in the pancreas. But in which part?

By Minkowski and Mering's day it was already understood that the pancreas was an organ of digestion that – to use modern language – synthesises the enzymes that digest the proteins, fats and carbohydrates in the diet. The enzymes are secreted into a duct that conveys them into the intestines, where they break down the food. But even before Minkowski and Mering had performed their experiment, a German doctor named Paul Langerhans (1847–88) had in 1869, while still a student, discovered that dotted throughout the pancreas were little 'islets' or collections of cells that appear under the microscope to be different from the mass of pancreatic cells. Unlike the other cells of the pancreas, the islets did not drain into a duct.

Langerhans didn't know what those islets did, but in 1893 the French scientist Edouard Laguesse suggested they might be the source of the anti-diabetic hormone we now call insulin. It's called that because it comes from Langerhans's islets. The word 'insular' has the same root.

(Langerhans died young, from tuberculosis, probably contracted from one of his patients. During the nineteenth century many doctors – including the great René Laennec, who invented the stethoscope – caught tuberculosis from their patients. The practice of medicine still carries its infective risks, as the deaths of doctors, nurses and other health workers during the recent Ebola outbreaks have shown.)

The next – key – advance came in 1921 when a young surgeon called Frederick Banting (1891–1941) led a small group at the University of Toronto that discovered how to isolate insulin. Banting's experiment was inspired. The obvious way of testing Laguesse's idea, that the islets secreted an anti-diabetic hormone, would have been to extract some pancreas, homogenise it, and then inject the homogenate into a patient with diabetes. But the pancreas synthesises a vast quantity of enzymes that digest proteins, and insulin is a protein, so preparing a homogenate of pancreas would destroy the insulin before it could be injected. Yet Banting knew that when the duct of an exocrine gland happens, for whatever reason, to get blocked, then the gland – under the backpressure – atrophies. In his words: 'In the first experiments, this was done by taking advantage of the fact that the acinous tissue (from which the digestive enzymes are derived) but not the insular tissue of the pancreas degenerates in seven to ten weeks after ligation of the pancreatic ducts.'[3]

Soon Banting was ligating the ducts of dogs, and soon those dogs were yielding pancreases that were free of the enzymes that digest proteins but whose islets were intact, which meant that those pancreases could be homogenised without instantly destroying their insulin. So it was that, on 11 January 1922, a 14-year-old boy called Leonard Thompson became the first person to be injected with a pancreatic extract containing insulin.

Thompson had been admitted with type 1 diabetes to the General Hospital in Toronto where he was expected, routinely, to die. Yet on 20 February that 14-year-old boy walked out of the hospital. Leonard Thompson's Lazarus-like walk represented one of the high dramas in western medicine (comparable to the drama generated in Oxford on 12 February 1941 when Florey and Chain injected their first patient, a 43-year-old policeman named Albert Alexander, with penicillin)[4] and a year later, in 1923, Banting and his colleague Macleod received the Nobel Prize. In keeping with Alfred Nobel's instructions, the prize was awarded promptly in those days.

Research success, group unhappiness

One unexpected aspect of science is that success can sometimes lead to unhappiness. When research groups struggle, the different members of a group will often unite in the face of adversity, but when successful those same researchers can fall out over the division of credit.

Frederick Banting was a remarkable man who won, for example, the Military Cross for gallantry in the First World War, but Banting resented the decision of the Nobel committee to divide his prize with Professor John Macleod (who was the head of department, and who had spent the key summer of 1921 salmon fishing on Skye, in Scotland) rather than with Charles Best, his principal colleague at the bench. Banting felt that Macleod had not made a sufficient contribution to the project to justify his sharing the prize, while the committee judged that, had Macleod not supported the project, it would not have succeeded.

Banting and Macleod were both admirable people (they donated, for example, their insulin patent to the University of Toronto, which used the royalties to fund further research), but Banting made public his rage by pointedly sharing his money from the prize with Best. Macleod responded by sharing his with James Collip, the biochemist who was the fourth member of the team. Banting's public rage with Macleod had enriched Best and Collip yet it had also diminished both leading protagonists. Sad. (See M. Bliss (1982), *The Discovery of Insulin*, McLelland and Stewart, Toronto.)

A definition: Before reviewing the research highlights that have flowed since the isolation of insulin in 1921, let me provide a definition of diabetes. Here is the one supplied by the American Diabetes Association: 'Diabetes mellitus is a group of metabolic diseases characterized by hyperglycemia [high levels of blood glucose] resulting from defects in insulin secretion, insulin action, or both.'[5]

There are two major types of diabetes mellitus, the rarer type 1 and the commoner type 2, but regardless of their differences, their shared characteristic of high blood levels of glucose means that they also share certain complications, namely that high blood glucose levels will gradually destroy the eyes, kidneys and small blood vessels.

Two types of diabetes mellitus: As early as the fifth century AD (CE) in his *Sushruta Samhita*, Sushruta, the Father of Indian Surgery, described two types of diabetes mellitus: 'Sweet is the urine . . . This disease may be ascribed to two causes, the congenital and that attributable to an injudicious diet . . . The former type is associated with emaciation, the latter with obesity and an inclination for lounging in bed or on cushions.'[6]

But Sushruta's insight never reached the west, and it was only in 1951 that R.D. Lawrence, who was the London physician who had jointly founded the Diabetic Association, (re)discovered the two types, recognising that type 1 (Sushruta's type that 'is associated with emaciation') was characterised by an absence of circulating blood insulin, while type 2 (Sushruta's type that is associated 'with obesity and an inclination for lounging in bed or on cushions') was characterised by its presence.

Some 5 to 10 per cent of diabetics are type 1. Some people still refer to type 1 by its old name of 'insulin dependent diabetes' and to type 2 as 'non-insulin dependent diabetes', and there's not much wrong with those old terms except that – with the increasing recognition of unusual subtypes of diabetes – we should probably stick to the terms 'type 1' and 'type 2' for the two major forms of the disease. I shall be saying nothing more about the unusual subtypes.

Type 1 diabetes: Type 1 diabetes is caused by the destruction of the insulin-secreting cells in the islets of Langerhans. Oddly, they are destroyed by the patient's own immune system.[7] No one knows why. Perhaps a passing virus confuses the immune system into killing the islet cells by accident (stranger things can happen in biology), but for our purposes we need know only this: in type 1, the insulin-secreting cells of the islets of Langhans die. Type 1 diabetes, therefore, is a disease of insulin deficiency. If we understand what insulin does, therefore, we will equally well understand type 1.

Understanding insulin: To understand insulin, let's start with some simple biochemistry. Einstein apparently said that every description in science should be made as simple as possible but no simpler, yet this section is legitimately simple.

As everybody knows, there are three major food groups, namely fats, proteins and carbohydrates. We all know what fat looks like, we can all recognise a steak, and we all know that carbohydrates come either in complex forms such as pasta or in simple forms such as sugar.

When we eat, our guts – thanks to the enzymes the pancreas has secreted into them – digest the three major groups down to their simple forms. So fats are broken into fatty acids and cholesterol, proteins are broken into amino acids, and carbohydrates are broken into sugars. The guts are well supplied by blood and lymphatic vessels, and on digestion these simple forms diffuse into the bloodstream. Insulin's job is to handle one of those forms, the sugar we call glucose (from *glykys*, the Greek word for 'sweet').

Glucose is a major fuel: starch is made up of long chains of it, and most people eat a lot of starch in the form of potatoes, bread, cereals, rice or pasta. Glucose, moreover, is a major component of household sugar, and many people consume a lot of that too. At least a third of our diet, therefore, generally breaks down into glucose, so insulin's handling of it is important.

Glucose being a fuel, the body's cells need to burn it, as cars burn petrol.* Yet the cells face a problem. If they are to burn glucose they will need to ingest it, but glucose is water-soluble whereas the membranes of the cells are composed of oily molecules, and we all know that oil and water do not mix. Glucose, therefore, can enter the cells of the body only through special

---

* The burning of glucose by the cells is indeed analogous to the burning of petrol in a car: the carbon and the other elements of the glucose bond with oxygen ('oxidation') to release carbon dioxide and other products including, of course, energy. The energy from the burning of petrol is released crudely, whereas the energy from the oxidation of glucose by the cells of the body is harnessed more subtly by sophisticated biochemical mechanisms, but the fundamental chemistry of oxidation is the same in both cases.

channels that penetrate the membranes. And there is a further complication: those membrane channels are not always open. Indeed, they are often closed. Which introduces insulin. Its job is to open those channels, which – in turn – means that the islets' job is to respond to raised levels of glucose in the blood by secreting it.

So when we absorb glucose from the guts into the blood-stream, the islets of Langerhans detect it, they secrete insulin – also into the bloodstream – and the insulin and the glucose then travel together to the cells of the body, where insulin opens the channels by which glucose enters the cells.

Once the glucose has been abstracted by the cells of the body, its levels in the blood will then fall. That fall will be detected by the islets, which will cease to secrete insulin, and the fall in the level of circulating insulin will, by default, lead to the closure of the glucose channels. Those closures will ensure that circulating blood levels of glucose do not fall much below 4 mmol/l, which as we'll see below is important for the protection of the brain.

FIGURE 17.1
24-hour pattern of insulin secretion

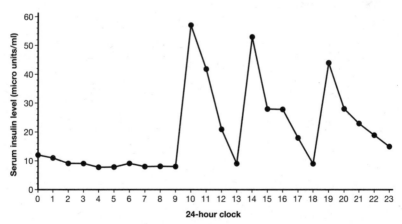

Typical levels of serum insulin in healthy people eating three typical meals a day at 9.00, 13.00 and 18.00. In people who are obese, the resting and post-prandial levels of insulin are at least double.

The daily pattern of insulin secretion: For obvious reasons, the daily pattern of insulin secretion mirrors that of blood glucose, rising after meals and falling between them.[8] To summarise, therefore, when we eat sugars and starches:

1 They are digested in the gut into glucose and other simple sugars
2 Which then diffuse into the bloodstream
3 The glucose in the blood is detected by the islets of Langerhans
4 Which then secrete insulin
5 Which travels in the bloodstream to the cells of the body
6 Where it opens their glucose channels
7 Which allow the glucose to enter the cells
8 And to be burned as a fuel.

Understanding type 1 diabetes: If those are the roles of insulin, it's not difficult to understand type 1 as a disease of insulin deficiency.

Without insulin, the glucose that is absorbed into the bloodstream from the gut after a meal has nowhere to go because there is no insulin to open the glucose channels in the cells of the body. So the glucose accumulates in the blood until eventually – when its levels exceed some 10 mmol/l – it spills into the urine: the job of the kidneys is to remove unwanted chemicals from the bloodstream, and glucose in high concentrations is an unwanted chemical.

But in type 1 diabetes the glucose is present in such high concentrations that, once in the urine, it provokes an osmotic effect that stimulates the excessive peeing that originally gave the disease its names of diuresis/diabetes. That peeing in its turn dehydrates the patient, who in consequence is soon driven by a violent thirst to drink compulsively: 'The patients never stop making water and the flow is incessant . . . The patients' thirst is unquenchable, their drinking is excessive.' Within a short time, therefore, of the destruction of their insulin-secreting cells, the type 1 diabetic presents today just as they did 2,000 years ago, namely with excessive thirst and excessive peeing.

The patient, moreover, starts to lose weight as the body suffers from the loss of glucose as a fuel: ironically, in type 1 diabetes there is glucose glucose everywhere nor any grain to burn, because the bloodstream is brimful of it yet it can't enter the cells. So, to find alternative fuels, the body breaks down muscle mass and fat mass into amino acids and fats, which – despite the absence of insulin – can be absorbed by tissues from the bloodstream and then oxidised. Yet those are desperate measures because, without insulin, the muscles and fat cells cannot replace the proteins and fats they have mobilised, so that way lies starvation unto death: 'a melting down of the flesh and limbs into urine . . . and within a short time they expire.'

The treatment of type 1 is unequivocal: insulin. Before Banting and Best discovered insulin, patients with type 1 died within a short time of diagnosis. Now, thanks to their discovery, type 1 diabetics can expect to live long and effective lives even though, unfortunately, their lives may not yet be as long or as complication-free as those of non-diabetics: a 2015 study of some 25,000 patients in Scotland concluded that the life expectancy of male type 1 diabetics is eleven years shorter than their peers, while for women the loss of years is even greater, at thirteen years.[9] As Banting said in his Nobel acceptance lecture of 15 September 1925: 'Insulin is not a cure for diabetes; it is a treatment.'[10] Yet the rate of advance in this field is heartening and we can anticipate ever better outcomes in the future.

18

Diabesity, the big new disease

For over a century people have understood that diabetes can be precipitated by overeating, which in turn can kill by precipitating cardiovascular catastrophe. In 1901, in his novel *Buddenbrooks*, Thomas Mann described the death of a north German patriarch:

> James Mollendorpf, the oldest of the merchant senators, died in a bizarre way. The instinct of self-preservation had weakened in this diabetic old man, and in the last years of his life he gorged on cakes and pastries. Dr Grabow, the family physician, protested, and the distressed relatives tried to dissuade the head of the family from committing suicide by confectionery. To evade his relations' entreaties, the old senator rented a room in a run-down part of town, far from his usual respectable haunts – a little hole of a room where he could eat sweets and pies and tarts in secret. And there they found his body, his mouth full of half-masticated patisserie. A stroke had accelerated his slow dissolution.

Type 2 diabetes is a different disease from type 1. Although it can present like type 1, with Arataeus's 'patients [who] never stop making water' and whose 'thirst is unquenchable', its causes are different, which is why it appears in Sushruta's people 'with obesity and an inclination for lounging in bed or on cushions'. So type 2 diabetes – rather than being an autoimmune disorder – owes more to the overeating that Thomas Mann described in

Buddenbrooks. And whereas circulating blood levels of insulin are low in type 1, in type 2 they can be . . . high! How can this be?

The clue lies in today's epidemic of obesity, which has emerged alongside today's epidemic of type 2 diabetes. The world today is in the grip of these two linked epidemics – indeed they are so linked that some scientists now talk of a disease called 'diabesity'. Let me provide some statistics, using data from the USA and the UK as representative of the industrialised nations, and using data from the World Health Organization (WHO) to provide a global overview.

The epidemiology of obesity: Obesity was once unusual but is now so common that in 1997 the World Health Organization formally recognised it as a global epidemic.[1] For obvious reasons an individual's obesity cannot be measured solely by their weight, so it is measured by the Body Mass Index (BMI) which uses a simple formula to correct for different people's heights.* See Table 18.1 over the page.

The BMI definitions were not selected arbitrarily: the World Health Organization has found that, for every point above 25 or below 18.5, a person's risk of dying or falling ill increases.[2] So, for example, people with a BMI greater than 35 have a hundredfold greater chance of developing type 2 diabetes than

---

* The formula is Body Mass Index (BMI) = weight in kilograms/height in metres squared (BMI = weight/height^2). To translate these figures into familiar ones, for a person of height 5'8":

Weight in stones	weight in kg	BMI
9.25	60	18.5
11.5	72.5	25
13.8	88	30
18.5	117	35

Every rise by one unit of BMI is approximately equivalent to a rise of half a stone or 3.5 kg in weight, though these relationships are not strictly linear.

Note that a raised BMI needn't reflect excess fat – in the super-fit it can reflect excess muscle – but on a population basis it correlates well with fat.

TABLE 18.1

BMI (kg/m², i.e. weight per height squared)

Figure	Description
Less than 18.5	Underweight
18.5 to 25	Normal
25 to 30	Overweight
30 to 35	Moderately obese
35 to 40	Severely obese
Over 40	Very severely (morbidly) obese

do normally weighted people,[3] and a reduced life expectancy by six to seven years.[4] But with every kilogram of weight lost by dieting, the risk of developing type 2 falls by 16 per cent.[5]

A too-low BMI also reduces life expectancy, and there is a so-called 'U shape' of mortality risk, with danger rising on either side of an optimal BMI at the 'bottom' of the U. That U shape has long been recognised, and in the *Merchant of Venice* (1596/97) Shakespeare's Nerissa says that: 'They are as sick that surfeit with too much as they are that starve with nothing' (Act 1, Scene 2).

In Shakespeare's day, of course, the perennial concern was the 'starve with nothing', whereas today it is the 'surfeit with too much' that has helped render a third of all adults worldwide overweight or obese.[6] So in the USA, for example, body weights rose on average by 24.4 pounds (1¾ stones or 11 kg) between the early 1960s and 2000, and though average heights also increased by about an inch (2.5cm), the increase in mean BMIs for adults from around 25 to around 28 showed that most of the extra mass went round, not up.[7]

Today there are more obese (not just overweight – obese) than underweight people globally,[8] and on current trends a fifth of all adults, globally, will be obese by 2025. The most acute obesity problems are to be found in certain emerging countries: in Tonga, for example, over half of all adults are obese (not just overweight – obese) while adults in certain other countries including Kuwait, Libya, Qatar and Samoa are almost as obese.[9]

But if only because of their greater populations, the greatest problems are to be found in the industrialised world, which certainly has its problems: every day in the UK two people on average have to be rescued by firefighters and paramedics after they have become stuck in their homes.[10] Windows as well as doors sometimes need to be taken out.

The five industrialised countries with the highest rates of overweight and obesity in 2012 were:[11]

Country	Overweight	Obese	Overweight and Obese
	%	%	%
Mexico	39.5	30.0	69.5
United States	33.3	35.9	69.2
United Kingdom	36.7	26.1	62.8
Australia	36.7	24.6	61.2
Canada	35.8	24.2	60.0

Because of the increased risks of heart attacks and strokes,[12] obesity appears to account for about 300,000 excess deaths per year in the USA alone,[13] second only to tobacco as a cause of excess deaths, and costing America $147 billion annually in medical costs.[14] In the case of Britain, McKinsey & Company, the management consultants, estimate that in 2012 obesity cost the UK economy £47 billion ($70 billion; 3 per cent of national GDP) in terms of health care and lost productivity, which was second only to smoking (at 3.6 per cent of GDP) as a self-inflicted burden. Internationally, McKinsey estimate that obesity (at 2.8 per cent of global GDP) is humanity's third-greatest self-inflicted burden, behind only smoking (2.9 per cent of global GDP) and armed violence/war/and terrorism (2.8 per cent of global GDP).[15]

Not all economies have yet emerged into industrialisation and, sadly, underweight remains a problem internationally (some 20 per cent of children are underweight globally). We thus face the paradox that, as the economies of the emerging world develop, so their populations may lurch from inadequate eating to reckless eating, with no period of moderation in the middle.[16]

The epidemiology of type 2 diabetes: Diabetes is showing similar trends to obesity. By 2012, 29.1 million Americans had been diagnosed with it, with another 8 million or so not having yet been diagnosed (many early diabetics go undiagnosed), meaning that some 9.3 per cent of the population had diabetes.[17] Since, in 2010, 'only' 25.8 million Americans had been diagnosed with diabetes, its incidence had risen from 8.3 per cent to 9.3 per cent of the population in just two years. Yet in 1960 less than 1 per cent of the American population had diabetes.[18]

Diabetes has become the seventh leading cause of death in the United States: in 2010, 234,051 death certificates listed it as an underlying or contributing cause of death[19] out of a total of 2,215,458 deaths that year.[20] The American Diabetes Association has calculated that the total cost of diagnosed diabetes in the United States in 2012 was $245 billion ($176 billion for direct medical costs and $69 billion in reduced productivity). And because Americans are continuing to live longer (the incidence of diabetes increases with age) and because Americans are becoming ever less Anglo-Saxon (many ethnic groups are more susceptible than Anglo-Saxons to diabetes) and because Americans remain too sedentary (exercise helps prevent diabetes) and because Americans are still overeating, the Centers for Disease Control and Prevention (CDC) extrapolate that, by 2050, some 20 to 33 per cent of Americans will be diagnosed with diabetes. The situation in America is now so worrying that on 29 October 2010 President Barack Obama proclaimed November to be National Diabetes Month, and he and his wife Michelle urged Americans to exercise more.*

---

* Someone who took Obama's proclamation seriously was his Democratic predecessor in the White House, Bill Clinton. After a quadruple heart bypass and the insertion of two coronary stents, Clinton so

Diabetes is also a major problem in Britain. In 2016 Diabetes UK reported that 4.05 million people (6 per cent of the population, including an estimated 549,000 people who have yet to be diagnosed*) suffer from it, accounting for some 24,000 premature deaths every year and, at £14+ billion annually, for some 10 per cent of the budget of the National Health Service.[21] But worse is to come, and in the words of Diabetes UK the number of people with type 2 'is set to rise dramatically over the next ten years'.[22]

And – again like obesity – diabetes affects the industrialising as well as the industrialised countries: in 2012 the World Health Organization found it to be the eighth leading cause of death globally. One of today's great joys is that wealth, globally, is rising fast, particularly in many formerly poor regions, but the worm in the apple is that, as the world's economies develop, their incidence of diabetes rises even faster. In the WHO's words: 'diabetes caused 1.5 million deaths in 2012 (2.7% of all deaths) up from 1.0 million (2.0%) in 2000.'[23]

The International Diabetes Federation estimates that by 2030 there will be 438 million diabetics worldwide (up from 285 million in 2010),[24] and the global situation is now so worrying that on 20 December 2006 the General Assembly of the United Nations designated 14 November as World Diabetes Day.

The epidemiology of overeating: The sudden rise in the incidence of obesity and diabetes cannot be attributed to a

---

intensified his interest in diet that in March 2014 his daughter Chelsea described him as 'probably the world's most famous vegan'. Apparently, though, his veganism is not total, and he is conflicted over fats – though not over sugar, which he knows to be bad (Sam Apple 15 May 2014, 'A mutable feast', *New Republic*, www.newrepublic.com/article/1177 76/bill-clintons-vegan-not-diet-proves-hes-baffled-we-are).

* The average patient with type 2 diabetes has had the condition for between four and seven years before it is diagnosed (M.I. Harris et al. (1992), 'Onset of NIDDM occurs at least 4–7 yr before clinical diagnosis', *Diabetes Care* 15: 815–19).

genetic change – such a change would take many generations
to express itself. The rise must be environmental in origin, and
the obvious cause is that we are overeating. That overeating
seems – if we can believe the evidence of western art – to have
been accelerating over a millennium. The Last Supper has long
been an iconic subject for painters, and in 2010, in an unusual
interdisciplinary collaboration, two brothers, Brian Wansink of
the Cornell University Food and Brand Laboratory, and Craig
Wansink who teaches religious studies at Virginia Wesleyan
College, published a paper in the *International Journal of Obesity* chronicling the size of the portions painted in fifty-two Last
Suppers between AD 1000 and AD 2000. They found that, over
the last thousand years, the size of portions has risen by 69 per
cent, the size of the plates by 66 per cent, and the size of the
accompanying pieces of bread by 23 per cent.[25]

Some art historians have criticised the Wansinks' study,[26] and
they have suggested that the evidence of the paintings can be
interpreted differently, but Brian Wansink nonetheless asserts
that, 'the last thousand years have seen dramatic increases in
the production, availability, safety, abundance and affordability
of food'[27] and that consequently we eat more than ever before.
He's of course right.

Overeating in the USA: The Centers for Disease Control and
Prevention (CDC) have reported that, in the thirty years between
1971 and 2000, American women increased their average daily
calorie intake by 22 per cent,[28] from 1,542 calories a day to
1,877.(the reference range for sedentary middle-aged women is
1,600–1,800 calories a day)[29] while men increased their average
daily calorie intake by 7 per cent from 2,450 to 2,618 calories
a day (the reference range for sedentary middle-aged men is
2,000–2,200 calories a day) so we can see that many Americans
are consuming too many calories.*

---

* These reference ranges are lower than those given in Box 1 in Chapter
1, because those assumed that people were taking a moderate amount
of exercise.

FIGURE 18.1

Obesity and the consumption of different foods 1960–2000 USA

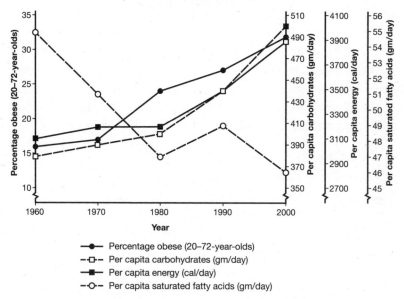

- —●— Percentage obese (20–72-year-olds)
- --□-- Per capita carbohydrates (gm/day)
- —■— Per capita energy (cal/day)
- --○-- Per capita saturated fatty acids (gm/day)

Between 1960 and 2000, the consumption of fats in the USA fell and the consumption of carbohydrates rose in response to the official dietary advice, which coincided with a rise in the rates of obesity and type 2 diabetes.

Dr Shi-Shen Zhou from Dalian, PR China, looking at the USA between 1950 and 2005, showed that the increase in obesity over that fifty-five-year period (from 14 per cent of the population to 33 per cent) correlated tightly with the increase in calorie intake. In turn, that correlated with the increase in the consumption of carbohydrates. At the same time, however, the consumption of meat, animal fats and cholesterol *fell* in response to the public health messages (Figure 18.1). Indeed, it's almost impossible from Zhou's paper to avoid the conclusion that it is the intake of carbohydrate rather than of fat that determines the incidence of diabetes and obesity in the USA.*

---

* Zhou believes that the niacin that is added to carbohydrate foods rather than the carbohydrates themselves may be the villain in terms

There are a number of mechanisms by which the carbo-hydratisation of our diets may have caused obesity and I discuss them shortly (clue: carbohydrates put us into a 'scoffin' kinda mood' in Robert Crampton's words, see p. 154), but let me note that it was around 1980 that the rates of increase in overweight and obesity in the USA accelerated,[30] so let us ask what changed around then. That must of course be a complex topic, and though it is surely no coincidence that the US federal government issued its first pro-carbohydrate health message in 1977, we can identify other factors as well, including:

- the falling price of food
- processed food and the burger wars
- the Snackwell effect
- grazing
- culture
- the market
- fat shaming
- denial
- exercise
- the Australian and British paradoxes.

The falling price of food: Food has become ever cheaper: in 1900 the average American spent 43 per cent of household income on food, but by 2003 that was down to 13 per cent.[31] Unfortunately, though, the cost of healthy foods such as fruit and vegetables may be rising, globally, while the cost of processed foods may be falling. In the UK, for example, the price of fresh green vegetables rose by 199 per cent in real terms between 1980 and 2012, while the price of an ice cream halved.

---

of diabetes and obesity: I find that idea improbable but in the interests of balance I reference it here (S.-S. Zhou et al. (2015), 'High serum N^1-methylnicotinamide in obesity and diabetes: a consequence of excess nicotinamide?', *J Clin Endocrinol Metab*, doi: 10.1210/jc.2015–711; and S.-S. Zhou et al. (2015), 'Management of nicotinamide N-methyl-transferase overexpression: inhibit the enzyme or reduce nicotinamide intake?', *Diabetologia* 58: 2191–2).

In Brazil, China, Mexico and South Korea, the price of fruit and vegetables rose by 99 per cent between 1980 and 2012, while some processed foods such as ready meals dropped in price by some 20 per cent.[32]

Processed food and the burger wars: No one who has read Eric Schlosser's 2001 book *Fast Food Nation* needs doubt that fast, junk and processed foods are bad for us, and Carlos Monteiro of the University of São Paulo, Brazil, has noted that: 'Production and consumption of ultra-processed food and drinks has sharply risen, especially since the 1980s . . . and supply most of the calories consumed in various high-income countries including the USA and UK.'[33]

Of the processed foods, few are more ubiquitous than hamburgers, and the late 1970s/early 1980s inaugurated the so-called 'burger wars' when McDonald's, Burger King, Wendy's and others started to carpet-bomb humanity with their fast foods, which are not only innately unhealthy but which seem to induce a 'kick' or 'high' not so different from that stimulated by certain addictive mood-altering chemicals.[34] Indeed, as Michael Moss reported in his 2013 book *Salt Sugar Fat: How the Food Giants Hooked Us*, fast, junk and processed foods are carefully engineered to hit our 'bliss point',[35] and their consumers can talk like addicts: after eighteen days of eating only at McDonald's, Morgan Spurlock said at one point in the 2004 film *Super Size Me* he 'was feeling awful . . . sick and unhappy . . . Started eating; now I feel great.'

The cola and soft-drink wars, too, have pumped people with empty calories from sugar, and these wars have been fuelled by the increase in children's spending power. And it may be no coincidence that the consumption of one particular carbohydrate, namely high-fructose corn syrup, rose dramatically between 1970 and 1990.[36]

The Snackwell effect: American nutritionists describe the so-called Snackwell effect. Snackwells were the American cookies that, in response to the public health messages, were manufactured fat-free. But to sustain their taste, the cookies were made sugar-rich. Yet the fat-free marketing persuaded many consumers into thinking they were eating healthy cookies, so their consumption soared.[37]

Grazing: Something else changed around 1980, namely the frequency of eating: once upon a time we were told not to 'eat between meals', but Barry Popkin and Kiyah Duffey from the University of North Carolina, on studying some 36,000 adults from 1977, found that over the next twenty-five years the number of 'eating occasions' (meals plus significant snacks) per adult per day rose on average from 3.5 to 5, while the gap between eating occasions fell from 4.5 hours to 3.5 hours.[38] People are now grazing all day, which Popkin and Duffey deplored because they found that the more often a person ate, the more food that person consumed.

Popkin and Duffey recognised that some authorities recommend a grazing lifestyle, but they found that the pro-grazing research studies were not always well designed, and that the bulk of the evidence suggests that, actually, fasting and eating fewer meals are better for a person's health. Popkin and Duffey are particularly critical of the advice to diabetics to eat frequently: 'With respect to diabetes, there is an unofficial consensus in clinical care that consuming evenly spaced eating occasions throughout the day is better than major binging episodes, but there are few formal research results supporting these recommendations.' (And, confirming Popkin and Duffey's scepticism, Dr Hana Kahleova of Charles University, Prague, has shown that type 2 diabetics do better if they eat only twice a day; see later.)

Grazing and breakfast: The implications of Popkin and Duffey's work for breakfast are obvious. As the journalist Robert Crampton wrote in *The Times* on 1 December 2015, the:

> problem with breakfast . . . is that far from setting you up for
> the day, it simply acts as a trigger to carry on eating. Breakfast

apologists argue that it guards against grazing later in the morning. My experience contradicts this: the 8.00 am bowl of porridge is more likely to lead to the 11.00 am bag of crisps than is the 8.00 am nothing at all . . . breakfast serves to get you into a scoffin' kinda mood. Much better to hold out as long as possible on fresh air.

I discuss later the biochemistry that underpins breakfast's getting us into a scoffin' kinda mood, but let us not leave Crampton quite yet because he is good on cereals. In his article, which was headlined 'Breakfast: it's the most dangerous meal of the day', he wrote: 'Most cereals are chock-full of sugar . . . (Sugar Puffs come to mind, no beating about the bush there) . . . as for fruit juices . . . suffice to say, when my children were small, their equally little friends who were plied with juice spent a lot of time at the dentist.'

Culture: The rise of grazing reflects a shift in our culture, and cultures do indeed shift. Sometimes (sorry to sound like a Marxist determinist) they shift in response to technology. As Dervla Murphy put it in her entertaining 1968 book *In Ethiopia With a Mule*:

> As I trotted downhill I reflected that the modern machine age has dangerously deprived Western man of whole areas of experience that until recently were common to the entire human race. Too many of us are now cut off from the basic sensual gratifications of resting after violent exercise, finding relief from extremes of heat or cold, eating when ravenously hungry and drinking when the ache of thirst makes water seem the most precious of God's creations.[39]

Conservatives protest when cultures shift into self-indulgence, and over two millennia ago in his *Memorabilia* of *c.*370 BC/BCE, Xenophon quoted Socrates quoting the nymph Virtue when she berated Hercules for: 'eating before you are hungry, drinking before you are thirsty, employing cooks to add to the pleasure of eating, buying costly wines to increase the pleasure of drinking . . . titillating yourself with gratuitous sex with boys and girls . . .'

The Bible, of course, got there earlier, and Jeremiah 5: 26–8, in his usual cheerful way, chronicled God's warning: 'Among my people are wicked men . . . They are fat and sleek and there is no limit to their wicked deeds' (New Living Translation).

Gluttony was, therefore, one of the seven deadly sins that Pope Gregory I (*c.*540– 604) condemned, which Dante (1265– 1321) echoed in his *Divine Comedy* when he delivered gluttons to the third circle of hell.

The market: But sometimes cultures change in response to markets. In his 2014 book *Sapiens: A Brief History of Humankind* the fashionable historian Y.N. Harari condemned the market for today's consumerism:

> Most people in history lived under circumstances of scarcity. Frugality was thus their watchword . . . A good person avoided luxuries, never threw food away, and patched up torn trousers . . .
>
> [but] consumerism sees the consumption of ever more goods and services as a positive thing. It encourages people to . . . kill themselves slowly by overconsumption . . . Just see the back of a cereal box. Here's a quote from a box of one of my favourite breakfast cereals, produced by an Israeli firm, Telma:
>
>> 'Sometimes you need a treat . . . There are times when you have to watch your weight and times when you've just got to have something, right now! Telma offers . . . you, treats without remorse.'
>
> Throughout most of history, people were likely to have been repelled rather than attracted by such a text. They would have branded it as selfish, decadent and morally corrupt.[40]

And certainly the market has encouraged our appetites: it is often said that the British became more healthy with food rationing during the Second World War (though looking at the data I think it would be more accurate to say that there's no reason to believe the British became less healthy)[41] yet the war-time food rations were, by modern standards, meagre.* So the weekly meat/protein ration for an adult in 1943 was one egg, up to a pound of meat, 3 pints of milk, 4 ounces of bacon/ham and 3–4 ounces of cheese.[42]

Today, though, the market presses us to eat. Professor Susan Jebb, the Oxford professor of diet and population health, told *The Times* on 8 April 2016 that almost all obese people were desperate to lose weight, which they had gained not because of a 'collapse in willpower' but because of genes, aggressive mar-keting ('every television advertising break provides temptation') and easy access to cheap food ('every town centre crawls with fast-food outlets'). Professor Jebb went on to say, 'You need in some cases a superhuman effort to reduce your food intake. Is that their fault? I don't think it is.'

As we have already discussed, weight is hugely determined by our genes, and a Cambridge research group found that over-weight people, when presented with a buffet of food, seem poor at controlling their impulse to eat, which the researchers linked to two parts of their brain being thin,[43] and which thus led the researchers to suggest that overweight may be neurologically determined (and which suggests that the old trick of dieting by emptying the fridge of food may not be so silly). In that spirit of biological determinism, in 2014 the European Court of Justice ruled in *Fag og Arbejde v Kommunernes Landsforening* that obesity was a disability, against which it can be illegal to

---

* Though during both world wars there were marked falls in deaths from diabetes, which tracked the falls in the sugar ration (T.L. Cleave (1974), *The Saccharine Disease*, John Wright & Sons, Bristol, Chap-ter 7, Figure 6 [no page numbers in the web version] journeytoforever. org/farm_library/Cleave/cleave_ch7.html). The fall in diabetic deaths, though, did not track the falls in the carbohydrate ration, thus remind-ing us that we are dealing with complex phenomena and that obesity and diabetes deaths are not identical.

discriminate: in the words of the plaintiff in the case, obesity 'is not a lifestyle choice; it's just the way I am'.[44]

Fat shaming: Nutritionists argue, moreover, that fat shaming does not work. So, for example, a 2014 study from University College London on 3,000 adults showed that the 150 of them who had suffered discrimination for their weight such as:

- receiving poorer service in restaurants, shops or hospitals or by doctors
- people acting as if they are stupid
- being threatened or harassed, or being treated with less respect or courtesy

put on more weight over four years (0.95 kg, 2 pounds) than those who did not (who actually lost 0.7 kg, 1½ pounds).[45] This was reported by the *Daily Mail* on 11 September 2014 as 'Telling someone they're fat makes them eat MORE,' and by the *Daily Telegraph* as 'Fat shaming "makes people eat more".'

But the research paper was describing only an association, and the cause and effect might go the other way: i.e. perhaps only people who put on weight suffered discrimination. So fat shaming *may* be counterproductive but we need a more critical view of the evidence.

Denial: There is widespread denial: a 2012 UK survey of 657 obese people revealed that only 34 per cent of the women and 23 per cent of the men acknowledged they were indeed 'obese or very overweight'.[46] Parental denial is also real: a 2015 British survey of the parents of 369 children who were very overweight or obese found that only four of those parents recognised their children's condition.[47]

The situation seems to be similar in the USA, and a survey of over 3,000 parents found that 95 per cent of the parents of overweight children considered their children to be the right weight, while 78 per cent of the parents of obese children also believed their children to be the right weight.[48]

The sense of denial was captured by Chimamanda Ngozi Adiche in her 2013 novel *Americanah*:

> 'fat' in America was a bad word, heaving with moral judgement like 'stupid' or 'bastard', and not a mere description like 'short' or 'tall'. So she had banished 'fat' from her vocabulary. But 'fat' came back to her last winter, after almost thirteen years, when a man in line behind her at the supermarket muttered, 'Fat people don't need to be eating that shit,' as she paid for her giant bag of Tostitos. She glanced at him, surprised, mildly offended, and thought it a perfect blog post, how this stranger had decided she was fat. She would file the post under the tag 'race, gender and body size'. But back home, as she stood and faced the mirror's truth, she realized that she had ignored, for too long, the new tightness of her clothes, the rubbing together of her inner thighs, the softer, rounder parts of her that shook when she moved. She *was* fat.[49]

Exercise: Over the last fifty years people in the industrialised world have engaged in less exercise. The decrease has not come from reducing recreational exercise – which has actually increased slightly as more people go to the gym or field – rather, it has come from the huge decrease in energy we expend in routine daily tasks as, for example, more people drive rather than walk, or as they use machines and white goods to alleviate household chores.[50] Consequently people now expend 500–1,000 fewer calories a day in daily life than they did 100 years ago.[51]

As the service industries displace agriculture and industry, so work is now also less physically demanding; it has even been calculated that spending two minutes an hour sending emails rather than spending two minutes walking down the corridor to speak to a colleague causes 5 kg weight gain each decade.[52] I return to exercise again shortly.

The Australian and British paradoxes: Because the USA now dominates nutrition research, there is a tendency to see the USA as the diabesity 'norm', but in 2011 a nutritionist at the University of Sydney, Jennie Brand-Miller, wrote a startling paper with the title: 'The Australian paradox: A substantial decline in sugar intake over the same timeframe that overweight and obesity have increased', which confirmed that between 1980 and 2003 obesity increased markedly in the USA, UK and Australia. But whereas sugar intake rose in the USA over that time by 23 per cent, it fell by 16 per cent in Australia and by 5 per cent in Britain.[53]

This unexpected finding (we all now 'know' that dietary sugar causes obesity the way we once 'knew' that dietary fat did) reinforces the suggestion that it is the insulin-resistance of the metabolic syndrome, not sugar per se, that is today's Public Enemy Number 1, but at the time Brand-Miller's research prompted certain critics to accuse her of scientific misconduct: it can be hard to ascertain how much food people really eat, because

- people report their food intake inaccurately because they underestimate it
- and so much food is thrown away that the producers' data is only an approximate guide

so critics argued that Brand-Miller was using inaccurate data.[54] She has since of course been cleared of misconduct, but in any case she is not alone: the British Heart Foundation has for years been reporting falls in food intake in Britain. So between 1975 and 2010

- average daily calorie intake fell from 2,498 to 2,035
- average daily fat intake fell from 112 to 84 g

and between 2000 and 2010

- average daily sugar intake fell from 131 to 116 g.[55]

The consumption of other carbohydrate-rich foods also fell.

So between 1942 and 2010

- average weekly bread consumption fell from 1,718 to 634 g.
- average weekly potato consumption fell from 1,877 to 501 g.

No less august a body than the British House of Commons has struggled to understand these data (how are we eating less yet getting fatter?) and its Health Committee quoted distinguished researchers to suggest that: 'The paradox of increasing obesity in the face of decreasing food intake can only be explained if levels of energy expenditure have declined faster than energy intake.'[56]

But there is a second explanation lurking in the data, because the British Heart Foundation reports that between 1950 and 2009 our

- weekly intake of fruit juice increased from 7 to 300 ml

while between 1942 and 2010 our

- weekly intake of breakfast cereals rose from 23 to 133 g.

And when do we consume fruit juices and breakfast cereals?

Some good news: Perhaps because food intake in the UK is falling, and perhaps because more people are skipping breakfast, the rate of increase in overweight and obesity seems too to be plateauing. On studying some 370,000 children, a team from King's College London found that between 1994 and 2003 the incidence of childhood overweight and obesity rose from around a quarter of the population to a third, but over the next decade – between 2004 and 2013 – it rose by only half a percentage point.[57]

Since there is a correlation between childhood overweight/obesity and adult overweight/obesity, the hope is that eventually this stabilising among children will translate into a stabilising of the adult rates – though not, one trusts, at the current rate by which two-thirds of UK adults are overweight or obese.

Conclusion: To use Nassim Taleb's terminology,[58] the human body is not antifragile, it is fragile, and I fear that everybody lets it down: its appetites betray it, the food producers seduce it, governments issue misleading *Guidelines*, the academics pursue outdated paradigms, and to top it all, we're encouraged to eat a gratuitous and meretricious meal – breakfast – that only increases our intake of calories and carbohydrates. Those in turn translate into the insulin-resistance of the metabolic syndrome.

Controversy over BMI

It was Dr Flegal of the CDC who first noted that rates of increase in overweight and obesity in the USA accelerated around 1980, and in 2005 she threw another bombshell when, on surveying some 25,000 people for some twenty years, she found that people in the overweight category (BMI 25–30) did not have an increased mortality.[59] Flegal has not been alone in finding that being overweight (as opposed to obese) seems no longer to be dangerous, and at least two other research groups agree with her.[60] But why may the BMI story have changed?

Well, most BMI researchers do not agree with Flegal. On 1 January 2013 Dr Walter Willett, the head of the department of nutrition at the Harvard School of Public Health, told *USA Today* that Flegal's work was 'complete rubbish' because her methodology was so flawed. He reiterated to US National Public Radio that 'this study is really a pile of rubbish and no one should waste their time reading it.' Go on, Walter, tell us what you really think (what he really thinks is that Flegal failed properly to correct for smoking, age and the weight loss that accompanies sickness).[61] And a conference convened at Harvard to consider Flegal's work dismissed it, arguing she had omitted key data.[62]

Flegal, on the other hand, thinks that improvements in the treatment of blood fats and hypertension have lowered the risks of being overweight, which in turn have lowered the excess death rates from overweight and obesity from around 300,000 per year in the USA to some 110,000. She thinks, moreover, that scientists have buried unwelcome findings: 'Publication bias can potentially affect systematic reviews. Studies that find little or no association of overweight or obesity with mortality risk sometimes only mention these results in passing without providing details.'[63]

The public argument between Flegal and Willett was startling, but some researchers believe that both may be right – some researchers believe in the 'obesity paradox', which says that fat can be good as well as bad for you.

An obesity paradox? Everybody – even Flegal – agrees that being large will precipitate type 2 diabetes, cardiovascular disease and cancer; nonetheless, once your raised BMI has given you such diseases, it can apparently come to your rescue. Consider a Scottish study on 4,880 patients who underwent angioplasties (when catheters are threaded into the coronary arteries to clear atherosclerotic plaques), which found that overweight people were more likely than normally weighted or obese patients to survive the operation.[64]

So being overweight helps precipitate heart disease, yet once people are diseased, that self-same overweight helps them to survive it. A paradox indeed, one that even the British Heart Foundation, which is no friend to fat, reported in a preliminary study:

How Fat Can Help Fight Heart Disease

The fat surrounding our blood vessels can help fight heart disease and reduce the risk of a heart attack . . . the results may explain the medical mystery that people with a high BMI, signifying obesity, are actually more likely to live longer after a heart attack . . . the fat releases chemicals that minimise oxidative stress and help to prevent the development of coronary heart disease.[65]

So when Wallis Simpson said you couldn't be too thin or too rich, she may have been only half right; and when Kate Moss said that nothing tastes as good as skinny feels, she might not have fully considered the post-angioplasty survival rates of skinny people.

The controversy between Flegal and Willett shows how compli-cated nutrition research can be. Harvard and the CDC are two of the most respected research outfits on the planet, yet they can't agree on the simplest but most important propositions. And conflict-ing data continue to appear. A recent Danish survey, for example, claimed that people with high BMIs who lost weight experienced a higher death rate than if they'd stayed large (for further complexi-ties, please see the reference).[66]

Sometimes I despair of making sense of all the conflicting data, but I think the mass of evidence nonetheless suggests that (i) the healthiest BMI is indeed to be found within the conventional normal range of 18.5–25, and (ii) that larger people should diet down to that weight, as long as they exercise seriously while simultaneously eat-ing protein and thus maintaining their muscle mass.

———————

19

Insulin-resistance, the modern plague

If overeating led only to overweight and obesity, would we care? The poundage would be a bore to drag around, and it would strain our joints, but it would not be life-threatening. Yet unfortunately the tonnage is the least of the consequences of overeating. *The* big consequence is insulin-resistance, which will kill about a third of us.

Bizarrely, though we've known for over seventy-five years that most type 2 diabetics are obese or overweight, and though we've known for over seventy-five years that many obese or overweight people become diabetic,[1] and though we've known for over forty-five years that obese people, like type 2 diabetics, have higher blood levels of insulin,[2] hardly anyone has heard of insulin-resistance; yet its death rate can be compared to the death rates from the bubonic plague during the Black Death years of 1346–53. Admittedly, insulin-resistance does not kill as fast as did the *Yersinia pestis* bacterium, but it kills as surely. It is the modern plague.[3]

Yet the term 'insulin-resistance' seems so obscure. Can such obscurity really be the cause of so much illness? In *Brideshead Revisited* Cara says of Lord Marchmain that he is dying of 'some long word at the heart'; so, equally, many of us will indeed die of an obscure term. Humanity has been here before, and bacteria like *Yersinia pestis* were once obscure: Pasteur struggled to persuade people that microscopic germs could cause human-sized diseases, and correspondingly people today need to be persuaded that insulin-resistance is as dangerous, and that only when we grow to view breakfast cereals and orange juice the way we now view unpasteurised milk will we take a quantum leap into health.

Becoming resistant to insulin: The key to understanding the modern epidemics is that people overeat, and in particular that they eat too much carbohydrate, so in consequence they secrete excessive amounts of insulin into the bloodstream.

Here comes the central issue. Insulin, like glucose, is a water-soluble molecule, so it cannot pass through the oily membranes of cells. So if insulin is to regulate cells' function (such as directing them to take up glucose) it needs to finesse its inability to enter them, which it does by binding to specific receptors lodged on the surface of the cells' membranes. When insulin binds to its receptor, therefore, it is the receptor – not the insulin itself – that passes a message into the interior of the cell, which then activates the glucose channels and the other cellular mechanisms that metabolise the glucose. But here's the key problem, here's the cause of so much death and disability: when receptors are over-stimulated by an excessive exposure to their hormone, they can down-regulate their responses; it's as if the receptors and their responses go on strike to protect their tissues from over-stimulation. It's as if the receptors are children who, should their parents shout too often, learn to ignore the shouts.

And that's what happens with insulin. As Professor Ralph DeFronzo of the Texas Diabetes Institute has shown, when insulin levels rise for too long – even to quite modest levels, simply to the upper end of the normal range – the cells soon become resistant to it. They down-regulate their responses to it.[4] They go on insulin strike. They ignore the shouts.

Ideally, the owner of these insulin receptors (i.e. you and me) would respond to a strike by cutting down on their eating – and indeed the fat cells of a person who overeats will try to inhibit the overeating by secreting a hormone called leptin (from the Greek *leptos* for 'thin') which suppresses appetite. Yet as we know, we do not eat solely to satisfy our bodily appetite, we eat also to satisfy our social and psychological appetites, and the effects of leptin can be overcome by social cues.[5]

So if an overeater continues to overeat, the islets have no choice but to overcome the receptor strike by pouring out even more insulin, which – at least initially – will keep down the blood levels of glucose. Thus do the islets try to keep down the levels of circulating blood glucose, but thus too does the overeater embark on the road to insulin-resistance.

To summarise the stages on the road to insulin-resistance:

1 A person overeats, especially carbohydrates
2 So excessive amounts of glucose enter the blood
3 So they secrete excessive amounts of insulin into the blood
4 Initially the insulin successfully pushes the excessive glucose into the cells
5 But the raised levels of insulin promote resistance to it by the cells
6 So the islets respond by secreting even more insulin, which – at least initially – overcomes the cells' resistance: blood glucose levels thus remain normal even though insulin levels are raised.

Some insulin resistance may be useful: Our biology is not stupid, and insulin-resistance evolved to be useful. In the words of two distinguished diabetologists: 'in insulin-resistant states in which glucose transport is impaired, sensitivity to insulin's antilipolytic [pro-fat] effect is relatively preserved, resulting in maintenance or expansion of adipose stores.'[6] In other words, we evolved to feast-and-famine, so when we feast we develop insulin-resistance, which diverts our excessive glucose to the fat stores, which makes good biological sense. Only when we, er, 'forget' to famine does our insulin-resistance persist and thus become a problem.

Prediabetes: Once a person's blood levels of insulin are raised, they may provoke even more insulin-resistance, thus generating a vicious circle of ever greater insulin-resistance leading to ever higher levels of circulating insulin, which provoke ever greater insulin-resistance. That ever greater resistance can eventually lead to the insulin, however high its concentrations, failing to keep down the blood levels of glucose, which then rise above the normal range. Unfortunately, therefore, like Hogarth adding a further plate to his *Rake's Progress*, we have to add a seventh stage to our road to insulin-resistance:

7 Because of the ever higher levels of insulin, the cells become even more resistant to it, and eventually certain blood glucose levels start to rise.

This condition has a name, prediabetes, which is a slightly misleading term that implies that prediabetes is little more than a forerunner of diabetes when, regrettably, there is a lot more to it than that: prediabetes, being a condition of raised insulin levels, is a mass killer. Yet the numbers of people with prediabetes is extraordinary. In 2012 no fewer than 86 million adult Americans or 37 per cent of the population had it: 51 per cent of those aged 65 and older.[7] In Britain the incidence of prediabetes is of American proportions, and in 2011 it affected 35 per cent of the population (49 per cent of those aged over 40).[8] Its incidence, moreover, is growing at a faster rate than in America, having affected only 12 per cent of the UK population in 2003. Some countries do even worse: the prevalence of prediabetes among adults in China is 50.1 per cent.[9]

Failure of the islets: from prediabetes to (in some cases) diabetes: Prediabetes is the state of insulin-resistance that affects half of all older people, but despite its misleading name, it does not always progress to type 2 diabetes. Type 2 develops only when someone has insulin-resistance *and* when their islets start to fail. People who have robust islets can apparently maintain a state of prediabetes indefinitely, but people who inherit the genes for vulnerable islets will, in the face of insulin-resistance, develop type 2 diabetes: their islets – exhausted by having worked too hard for too long – will start to fail, and their rates of insulin secretion will start to fall, and so their blood levels of glucose will rise into the diabetic range.

It generally takes about ten to twenty years of overeating in the face of insulin-resistance for susceptible people to succumb to type 2 diabetes, so the islets do put up a fight,[10] but nonetheless, as the insulin levels in these people eventually start to decline from their previously very high levels, so the blood levels of glucose will start to rise out of the prediabetic range into the diabetic range.[11] Sadly, therefore, we have to add a final stage to the road of insulin-resistance:

8 If the islets of Langerhans start to exhaust themselves, their secretion of insulin will therefore decline, so circulating blood levels of glucose will rise into the diabetic range.

Remember, though, that while the raised blood glucose levels of diabetes are dangerous to diabetics, the mass population-wide killer is the raised insulin levels of insulin-resistance and prediabetes.

Type 2 diabetes

Insulin-resistance is the condition that breakfast aggravates, and is thus the object of this book. Type 2 diabetes, however, is not a central concern of this book, so I shall relegate a few essential facts about it to this section.

What causes type 2?: Type 2 runs in families, so we know it is a genetic disease. Yet we also know it is caused by overeating, so how does that work?

Well, the relationship between overeating and type 2 diabetes is like that between smoking and lung cancer: if we didn't smoke very few of us would develop lung cancer and, equally, if we didn't overeat very few of us would develop type 2 diabetes. Nonetheless, not every smoker develops lung cancer, and not every overeater develops type 2 diabetes; so to develop lung cancer, a person needs both to smoke and to inherit a genetic weakness and, correspondingly, to develop type 2 diabetes a person needs both to overeat and to inherit a genetic weakness.

We know that variations of at least forty different genes can prime type 2 diabetes,[12] but we don't yet know how they each act to give us the disease. We do know, however, of at least three major classes of defect, namely inherited insulin-resistance, islet failure and pancreatic fat.

Inherited insulin-resistance: One inherited weakness was revealed in 2003 by a Polish research team. The team recruited thirty-four lean healthy people, seventeen of whom had close relatives with type 2 diabetes, seventeen of whom had no such relatives (they had lots of relatives, just none with type 2). Both sets of seventeen people had

- normal fasting levels of glucose
- normal levels of HbA1c
- normal glucose tolerance tests

so on an ordinary visit to an ordinary doctor they would all have been pronounced healthy. But when the Polish team looked at circulating insulin, they found that the people with close diabetic relatives had markedly raised levels. That is to say, these close relatives had been born with insulin-resistance,[13] and it would presumably require relatively little overeating to push them into prediabetes, and from there into frank diabetes.

Islet failure: Other genes, however, prime islet failure. Professor Ralph DeFronzo from Texas found that, when he infused the fats called free fatty acids into healthy subjects, their insulin levels rose. But when he infused free fatty acids into healthy subjects who had relatives with type 2 diabetes, their insulin levels dropped.[14]

So the islets of type 2 diabetics appear to be prone to damage by raised levels of free fatty acids (and of glucose) and we no longer speak of islet 'exhaustion' but, rather, of 'lipotoxicity' and 'gluco-toxicity', which simply mean that the islets of type 2s are damaged by high levels of free fatty acids or glucose.

Pancreatic fat: Because abdominal fat cells release their fat into blood vessels that directly feed the liver, which is the body's great metabolic organiser, the abdomen provides a rational place in which to deposit fat during a feast in preparation for mobilising it during the next famine, hence today's epidemic of pot-bellies. But in 2015 Professor Roy Taylor of the University of Newcastle upon Tyne, UK, showed that, when someone deposits fat within their abdomen, they often also deposit it within their pancreas (which lies of course within the abdomen) and that person will develop type 2 diabetes.[15]

But if that person then loses weight by going on a diet, such that they lose their extra pancreatic fat, so too does their diabetes reverse. So pancreatic fat seems to be the causative mechanism of type 2 diabetes.[16]

Conclusion: Drs Straczkowski, DeFronzo and Taylor have each made major advances in our understanding of type 2 diabetes, and the challenge now is to integrate their work in one unified theory.[17]

20

Definitions

So far I've used the terms 'prediabetes' and 'type 2 diabetes' without describing how they are diagnosed within individual patients. In so doing I may seem to be moving away from breakfast, but I'm going to locate this chapter in our concerns over prediabetes and breakfast.

How to make a diagnosis: When I was at medical school I learned that a diagnosis is made by a sixfold process of:

- history (asking the patient what has happened)
- clinical examination, which consists of
  - observation (looking at the patient)
  - palpation (feeling the patient's body)
  - percussion (tapping at the patient's chest)
  - auscultation (using the stethoscope)
- special investigations (which include blood tests, X rays and biopsies).

Traditionally the British have placed greater emphasis than the Americans on the first five, clinical, stages than on the sixth, namely special investigations, and at medical school I was taught that after you'd taken a history you should already have a good idea of the diagnosis, and that special investigations were to be ordered only to confirm your differential diagnosis. But during the 1980s, when I was on sabbatical in Cleveland, Ohio, an American physician complained to me, loudly – within earshot of a ward full of patients – that 'You limeys think that medicine is about clinical skills. That's all crap. Medicine is a quantitative science.'

Well, this chapter is a homage to the American model of medicine, because the diagnoses of prediabetes and diabetes reduce largely to measurements of blood glucose levels.

Insulin-resistance: The measurement of insulin-resistance is complex, and it is normally performed only by researchers, so we do not measure it in routine practice, which is a shame as – even in the absence of raised levels of glucose – high insulin-resistance is dangerous. But it can in any case be guesstimated by an intelligent interpretation of blood glucose levels and a careful medical history. Everyone who is over forty-five, more-over, and who is unfit or who has a raised BMI, should assume they are insulin-resistant even if their glucose levels are normal, and they should eat and exercise accordingly.

Prediabetes: This is an 'in-between' diagnosis, so let me move on to the diagnosis of diabetes and then return to it.

Diabetes: This is a disease of raised circulating levels of blood glucose, so first we need to ask: what are the normal blood glucose levels? Let's start with the fasting levels.

When doctors determine fasting blood glucose levels, they traditionally test early in the morning because the overnight fast is not only the longest and thus most complete of the twenty-four-hour cycle, it is also the most trustworthy: it's hard for a peckish patient to cheat by eating a secret snack when they are asleep.

Conventionally, normal ranges in medicine are defined as the values within which 95 per cent of the healthy population fall, and from many observations the normal or reference ranges for fasting blood glucose levels are generally reported to be 3.9 to 5.5 mmol/l. Here, though, we are interested only in the top of the normal range, so that is what appears in Table 20.1.

TABLE 20.1
A blood glucose level

Fasting capillary blood glucose
Normal   Less than 5.6 mmol/l

This figure, like all the blood glucose figures in subsequent tables, comes from the American Diabetes Association as reported by Bilous and Donnelly in their 2010 *Handbook of Diabetes*.[1]

I have provided the blood glucose figure only for capillary blood, which is the fingerprick blood we can measure at home on our personal glucometers. The professionals, though, generally measure levels of glucose in blood that has been obtained from veins by venepuncture (i.e. via a syringe taken by a phlebotomist) and these different technologies generate slightly different normal ranges that, for completion, I provide in the reference,[2] but the differences between them are small.

Post-prandial blood levels: * Blood glucose levels rise after a meal: can we capture that phenomenon, to determine the normal blood glucose response to a meal? Obviously different meals contain different foods, but in the clinic we can administer a standard 'meal', namely a standard amount of glucose, to generate a test known as the 'oral glucose tolerance test' (OGTT). The term 'tolerance', with its overtones of allergy, may at first sight appear unhelpful, yet it is useful to think of diabetes as a disease of glucose *in*tolerance. Had the authorities remembered that, they would not have launched their decades-old advice to consume a lot of carbohydrates.

In the glucose tolerance test, subjects are fasted overnight and

---

* Medical terms generally have reasonably rational derivations, but 'prandial' is an exception. It derives from the Latin *prandium* which means 'a late breakfast or lunch', but today doctors and scientists use 'prandial' to refer to any meal or snack. So 'post-prandial' follows any ingestion of food.

then given a drink, often Lucozade (394 ml), containing 75 g glucose.* After drinking it, a person's blood glucose levels rise, but – in healthy people – they fall within two hours to below 7.8 mmol/l. Table 20.2 is the same as Table 20.1 except that I've incorporated the two-hour results of the OGTT.**

TABLE 20.2
Two blood glucose levels

Fasting capillary blood glucose

Normal	Less than 5.6 mmol/l

2-hour capillary blood glucose

Normal	Less than 7.8 mmol/l

Now comes some philosophy. What is diabetes? If the only diabetes was type 1 in young people, philosophy (or careful definitions) might be irrelevant: young people would either have normal levels of blood glucose or they would present to doctors with recent histories of excessive thirst, excessive peeing and weight loss that, on investigation, would be associated with very excessive levels of blood glucose indeed. There would be few grey areas outside the first few months of the disease (when some insulin-secreting cells survive, so preventing blood glucose levels from reaching stratospheric levels). Instead, however, prediabetes is amazingly common, and the dominant type of diabetes is type 2, so we inhabit a world of grey areas where lots of people fall outside the normal reference ranges. So are they all diabetic? Curiously, they are not.

The definition of diabetes is that it is a disease of hyper-

---

* In the USA, dosing is by weight, namely 1.75 g of glucose per kg body weight, up to a maximum dose of 75 g. Before 1975 the dose was 100 g.

** A glucose tolerance test is administered only when a diagnosis of diabetes is in doubt. I, who presented to my doctor with a blood glucose of 19.3 mmol/l, certainly didn't need a diagnostic test! But patients with signs and symptoms of diabetes or prediabetes, yet whose fasting glucose level runs below 5.6, might have their glucose tolerance tested.

glycaemia or of high levels of blood glucose – and who'd have thought it, but glucose is a deadly threat. Consequently, on top of their other problems with insulin, diabetics suffer from the specific complications of high circulating blood levels of glucose. Those, in turn, are the product of the chemical process known as glycation.

The specific complications of diabetes: glycation: When you toast a slice of bread, when you roast a chicken or when you fry potatoes, the surface of your foodstuff goes brown, which is because the sugars and proteins in the foodstuff bind to each other to create a compound that happens to be brown. That process of so-called 'glycation' occurs, in fact, whenever sugars and protein are in contact, but the process is hugely accelerated by the heat of cooking.

The process is also accelerated by high concentrations of sugar, even at body temperature. The blood, for example, is a swirling vat of sugars and proteins that positively invite glycation. Glucose thus binds to blood proteins such as haemoglobin to generate the well-known blood test of HbA1c (haemoglobin A1c). Since the rate of glycation depends on the concentration of glucose, the concentration of HbA1c provides a test of how well a patient is controlling their blood sugar levels: the higher the average level of glucose, the higher the level of HbA1c.

So what? Why should glycation matter? Which is another way of asking: do high blood glucose levels matter?

Well, both types of diabetes mellitus are characterised by similar complications caused by damaged *small* blood vessels or capillaries (damage to large blood vessels is the domain of insulin, damage to small blood vessels the domain of glucose). Those small blood vessel complications include (i) blindness (1,280 new cases of diabetic blindness are reported every year in the UK[3] and diabetes is the most common cause of blindness among working-age adults)[4], (ii) renal failure (11 per cent of type 2s die from renal disease)[5] and (iii) amputations (100 diabetic limbs are amputated every week in the UK).[6] The damage to the small blood vessels that leads to these terrible complications is caused by their glycation by the raised levels of glucose in the blood.

So, yes, raised blood levels of glucose are damaging.

Diagnosing diabetes: In diagnosing diabetes, therefore, doctors have sought to determine which blood levels of glucose are associated with the specific complications of the disease, and – because of its relative ease of quantification – the doctors chose the eye damage as the reference complication.[7] And clinical experience with long-established patients shows that the eye pathologies are not seen until glucose fasting levels routinely exceed 6.0 mmol/l, which has generated the international agreement to define diabetes by that level.*

Equally, diabetes is also associated with raised levels of blood glucose after a meal, and clinical experience with long-established patients shows that the complications of diabetes start to be seen when patients routinely demonstrate two-hour blood glucose levels in excess of 11.0 mmol/l. Table 20.3 chronicles these points.

TABLE 20.3
Fasting normal and diabetic blood glucose levels

Fasting capillary blood glucose

Normal	Less than 5.6 mmol/l
Diabetic	Over 6.0 mmol/l

2-hour capillary blood glucose

Normal	Less than 7.8 mmol/l
Diabetic	Greater than 11.0 mmol/l

---

* The World Health Organization uses different, higher, criteria. In its words: 'There are important differences between (i) defining diabetes to identify an individual with diabetes and . . . (ii) defining diabetes for epidemiological purposes' (WHO (2006), *Definition and Diagnosis of Diabetes Mellitus and Intermediate Hyperglycaemia*, WHO Press, Geneva, Switzerland).

Prediabetes (again): Which brings us back to prediabetes. If normality is defined as the blood glucose levels shown by 95 per cent of normal people, and if diabetes is defined by the fasting and two-hour levels that are associated with the eye complications of the disease, then between these two sets of levels there is a gap, which is named prediabetes. This is captured in Table 20.4, which displays all the data provided in Tables 20.1–3 and then shows how prediabetes fills the gap.

TABLE 20.4
Normal and diabetic blood glucose levels

Fasting capillary blood glucose

Normal	Less than 5.6 mmol/l
Prediabetic	Between 5.6 and 6.0 mmol/l
Diabetic	Over 6.0 mmol/l

2-hour capillary blood glucose

Normal	Less than 7.8 mmol/l
Prediabetic	7.8–11.0 mmol/l
Diabetic	Greater than 11.0 mmol/l

Completing the bookkeeping: If, on being randomly tested for blood glucose (i.e. the test is done at no particular time of day, nor with any particular reference to food), someone demonstrates a blood glucose level that exceeds 11.0 mmol/l, they are probably diabetic and will require further investigation.

Finally, the glycation of haemoglobin allows us to use it as a blood test, and because haemoglobin circulates in the bloodstream for months, glycosylated haemoglobin (HbA1c) provides an average assessment of blood sugar over those months. The reference ranges are:

- healthy if HbA1c is below 42 mmol/mol
- prediabetic if HbA1c is between 42 and 47 mmol/mol
- diabetic if HbA1c is above 48 mmol/mol (i.e. this is the level associated with an increased risk of eye disease).

Conclusion: With these definitions under our belts, we are now equipped to understand *how* breakfast wreaks its dangers.

21

The dawn phenomenon

I've shown that breakfast as a morning meal is dangerous, but I haven't explained the two mechanisms of that matitudinal danger. One of them is cortisol.

The circadian/diurnal rhythm: As everybody knows, we are subject to the workings of the circadian or diurnal rhythm (from the Latin *circa* meaning 'around', and *diem* or *dies* meaning 'day', and *diurnalis* meaning 'of a day'). Consequently, not all meal times are equal.

As everybody also knows, circadian rhythms are driven by the light/dark cycle. Specialised brain cells connected to the eyes recognise the rising and the setting of the sun, and those cells drive glands at the base of the brain to secrete hormones in a cyclical fashion. Those hormones in their turn regulate many of the circadian rhythms of the body: over 10 per cent of the active genes in the body oscillate during the day, and their oscillations are generally controlled by the hormones that are themselves controlled by the light-sensitive cells of the brain.[1] Figure 21.1 shows how the blood levels of two key hormones change – really quite dramatically – over the twenty-four-hour cycle.

The 'classic' diurnal hormone is melatonin. This hormone is secreted by the pineal gland, which is a tiny structure at the base of the brain. Descartes believed the pineal gland to be the seat of the soul, but we now recognise it as the central conductor of the light/dark circadian orchestra: its secretion of melatonin leads most of the body's circadian rhythms. During the day melatonin

FIGURE 21.1
24-hour levels of melatonin and cortisol

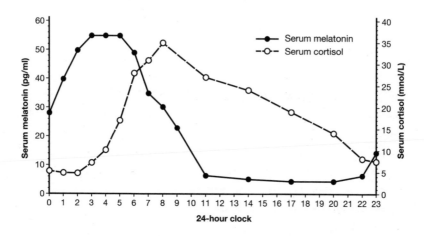

These are typical results from healthy young people.

levels in the blood are vanishingly small, but they peak between 2.00 and 4.00 in the morning, and the importance of melatonin is confirmed by its value in the treatment of jet lag. Jet lag arises because our diurnal rhythm has fallen out of sync with our new environment, and in the words of Cochrane, which is the most authoritative clinical auditing organisation on the planet: 'Melatonin [taken by mouth] is remarkably effective in preventing or reducing jet lag . . . it should be recommended to adult travellers flying across five or more time zones.'[2]

Melatonin appears to have no direct relevance to breakfast in diabetics, but there is another diurnal hormone, cortisol, that does. Cortisol is the 'alertness' hormone: its circulating blood levels rise in the early morning (thus helping wake us up) but its levels fall by the evening (thus allowing us to fall asleep). Its job is to reinforce a heightened sense of awareness.[3]

If cortisol only heightened our sense of alertness, breakfast might have evolved to be a safer meal, but cortisol has a second function, namely to be secreted during the so-called 'fight or flight' reaction: if we are to fight or flee a sabre-toothed tiger or a tribal enemy, we need to be alert, so when alarmed we secrete cortisol into the bloodstream – where it not only keeps us alert but also raises our circulating levels of blood glucose. Why?

Well, when fighting or fleeing, our muscles may need to burn glucose *fast* and, to mobilise that glucose, cortisol opposes the effects of insulin (insulin, of course, lowers blood sugar levels). Cortisol, therefore, induces insulin-resistance, which raises blood glucose levels and which – through non-insulin mechanisms – provides muscles with an urgent source of fuel.[4] But because cortisol is also secreted in the mornings, our mornings are characterised by a cortisol-induced insulin-resistance.

In their renowned if pompously titled 1979 essay, 'The spandrels of San Marco and the Panglossian paradigm: a critique of the adaptationist programme', Stephen Jay Gould and Richard Lewontin borrowed the term 'spandrel' from architecture to describe a biological feature that did not evolve in its own right but as a by-product of something else.[5] In architecture, spandrels are features that fill the gaps between arches and a dome: when an architect designs a dome to be supported by arches, they consequently create gaps between the dome and the arches. Those gaps needs infilling, and the fillers are called spandrels: but no architect, Gould and Lewontin argued, starts by designing spandrels; they design them only as a by-product of the arch/dome motif.

Equally, it's not clear if the glucose-raising property of cortisol in the morning has been selected by evolution as a good thing in itself, or if it is only a by-product of cortisol's alternative role as a fight-or-flight hormone, but either way our morning insulin resistance is real.

The dawn phenomenon: In the face of morning cortisol, it is no surprise that type 2 diabetics express the 'dawn phenomenon' of high blood glucose levels in the morning. Whereas the blood glucose levels of healthy people will fall overnight and will stay fallen, those of type 2 diabetics will, towards dawn, rise. So in chapter 1, describing Professor Christiansen's experiment, I noted that, whereas healthy people woke with morning blood glucoses of around 4–5 mmol/l, Professor Christiansen's type 2 diabetics woke with blood glucose levels of around 7.0 mmol/l.

Significantly, the extent of the dawn phenomenon correlates with the severity of the type 2 diabetes. So a study from the Diabetes Research Unit, Penarth, UK, showed that mild diabetics (HbA1c less than 7.3 per cent or 56 mmol/mol) wake with circulating blood glucose levels of about 7.0 mmol/l (rising to around 11.5 mmol/l after breakfast), while severe diabetics (HbA1c greater than 8 per cent or 64 mmol/mol) wake with circulating blood glucose levels of about 10.0 mmol/l (rising to around 15.0 mmol/l after breakfast).

What bewilders me about those findings is: *why, with those dangerously high post-breakfast blood glucose levels, were those patients eating breakfast at all?* But that's a question I shall address later. Here I want to ask: why does the morning blood glucose level in type 2 diabetics correlate with the severity of the disease? One answer is that diabetics possess a further glucose-raising factor in the morning called 'free fatty acids'.

Free fatty acids: When I became a medical student in the early 1970s, it soon became obvious that my peers' least favourite subject was biochemistry. Anatomy didn't frighten them because that required only that they learn long lists of facts, which medical students rarely seem to mind doing. Physiology (the science of bodily function) was positively interesting, and pharmacology reasonably so. But biochemistry? Yuk. Today it's apparent that, as medical students have become more academic, so they dislike biochemistry less, but I remain aware that biochemistry (the chemistry of bodily function) will never be universally loved, so I write the next few paragraphs with trepidation.

Here is the biological problem to which free fatty acids are the solution. As we all know, glucose is a major bodily fuel; it derives from carbohydrate, it circulates freely in the blood, and it is easily oxidised by our tissues. So of course glucose is a major fuel, but there is a worm in that apple – storage.

FIGURE 21.2

The relationship between triglyceride and free fatty acid

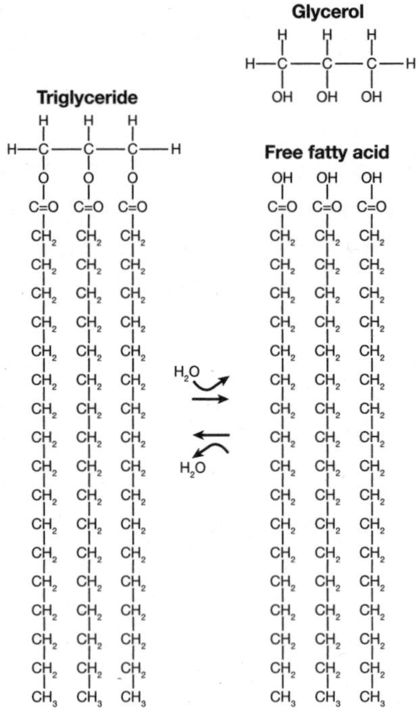

When insulin levels are high, triglycerides are stored in the fat cells.
But when insulin levels fall, the triglycerides are broken down into free
fatty acids and glycerol, which leak into the bloodstream and feed
the tissues of the body.

Glucose cannot be stored as a free chemical because it is soluble in water, and the amounts that can be dissolved in solution will power a cell for only a few seconds; fuel stores need to be solid so that they can be packed as dense reservoirs of energy. Glucose is therefore stored as glycogen (from *glykys* 'sweet' as in 'glucose' and *genes* as in 'Genesis' or 'birth'). Glycogen used to be known as 'animal starch' because, like its equivalent in plants (ordinary starch), it consists of long chains of glucose, bound together chemically. But glycogen is a poor fuel store. For two reasons.

First, being a carbohydrate, glycogen is already partly oxidised (the generic formula is CH_2O, hence 'carbo' and 'hydrate' because the C has been hydrated with H_2O) so the only energy it yields on oxidation comes from the oxidation of C to CO_2 or carbon dioxide: there is no energy to be released from the oxidation of H to H_2O because the H comes pre-oxidised.

The other problem is that glycogen is very water-friendly. It is, in itself, too big a molecule to be water-soluble, so it is stored as granules, but glycogen consists of glucose units that are innately very water-soluble, so in consequence much of the material that is stored in glycogen granules is actually water, whose molecules have inserted themselves within the glycogen molecules. Water is useless as a fuel but it occupies a lot of space and it weighs a lot, so the body can store only a few hours' worth of glycogen granules (in the liver largely).

Fat on the other hand makes a much better fuel store, for two reasons. First, its generic formula is CH_2, so its oxidation releases not only the energy of $C \rightarrow CO_2$ but also the energy from $H \rightarrow H_2O$. Further, fat is neither water-soluble nor water-friendly, so on storage it is not bulked by useless water. For these two reasons, therefore, it makes sense for the body to prioritise fat as a store of energy, which is why we store only some 900 calories of glycogen but up to 120,000 calories of fat in the form of triglycerides.[6]

But here comes the problem. When fat is released from the fat stores, it is released not as glucose but, reasonably enough, as fat – specifically, in the form of fat we call free fatty acids. So tissues need to be able to oxidise two different sources of energy:

- after a meal, tissues need to oxidise the glucose that comes from the gut
- but when we are fasting, tissues need to oxidise the free fatty acids that come from the fat stores.

This is what happens. It's a four-stage process.

- when meals are being digested, glucose passes from the gut into the bloodstream, where the islets of Langerhans detect it. So they secrete insulin, and the body's cells take up and oxidise the glucose

- but once a meal has been fully digested (which takes about four to six hours) no more glucose will pass from the gut into the bloodstream, so blood glucose levels will fall, which the islets will detect so they will reduce their release of insulin

- the lowering of insulin is itself a signal that directs the liver to break down glycogen and to release glucose into the bloodstream

- but the glycogen stores last only a few hours (by morning most of the liver glycogen has been exhausted by the overnight fast) so after a few hours' fasting, after the glycogen stores are exhausted, and after blood levels of insulin have fallen even further, those low insulin levels then act as a second signal: they direct the fat stores to release free fatty acids into the bloodstream.

In a rational world, a fasting body would first consume the glycogen-derived glucose and then, after the liver stores of glycogen had been exhausted, switch to oxidising free fatty acids. But the body is not so rational because the brain does not readily oxidise free fatty acids: it needs to continue oxidising glucose when the rest of the body has gone over to oxidising free fatty acids. Why? Nobody really knows. It's a mystery.[7]

But it's a mystery with consequences, because – when a body is fasting – its cells are thus presented with two fuels in the bloodstream: glucose (for the brain) and free fatty acids (for all the other tissues). Which is worrying, because 'ordinary' cells might consume the glucose that is rightfully the brain's. So, to ensure the other cells do not consume the precious glucose, they are signalled to understand that – if presented with both glucose and free fatty acids – they should consume only the free fatty acids, thus reserving the glucose for the brain.

And what signals the body's cells to consume only free fatty acids? The free fatty acids themselves, which induce massive, near-universal glucose- and insulin-resistance.[8] Which brings us back to breakfast and the dawn phenomenon.

Because free fatty acids are released when we are fasting, it is no surprise that circulating blood levels of free fatty acid levels are at their highest just before breakfast.[9] Consequently, the insulin-resistance they create will be at its highest at breakfast. So the free fatty acids' induction of insulin-resistance will reinforce the blood-glucose-raising effects of cortisol. That combination of high dawn levels of cortisol and of free fatty acids will tend to raise the dawn levels of glucose even in healthy people (though the insulin levels of healthy people will rise to accommodate the morning resistance), but in type 2 diabetes that insulin rise will not be enough to fully lower the blood levels of glucose.

In type 2, moreover, the insulin-resistance will weaken the fat cells' response to insulin, so they will release more free fatty acids, which will increase the insulin-resistance, so the blood glucose levels will be higher. It's a vicious circle – one that breakfast aggravates.

And the solution? Simple. Type 2 diabetics should skip breakfast. By lunchtime the diurnal dawn rise in cortisol will have fallen, and though the free fatty acid levels will still be high, they provide only one – not two – hurdles for the insulin to vault, and the empirical evidence is clear: in type 2 diabetes the insulin vaults the sole lunchtime hurdle much more easily than it does the double breakfast hurdle.

Some personalities

Writing this chapter sparked some memories I might perhaps share. First, the scientist who discovered that fatty acids displace glucose as a fuel was my own PhD supervisor, the eminent Professor Sir Philip Randle FRS. Philip called the phenomenon the 'glucose fatty acid cycle'. Unaccountably, Philip – having made this discovery –

was for some fifteen years thereafter excluded from the fellowship of the Royal Society, the club of top scientists, apparently because Hans Krebs, the legendary Nobel laureate who had described his own celebrated 'Krebs cycle', was so offended by the hijacking of his term 'cycle' that he barred Philip. And you thought scientists were rarefied beings of dispassionate reason?

When I was doing my PhD, my lab adjoined Krebs's – and Krebs was among those researchers who showed how, after a few days' fast, the liver starts to turn free fatty acids into ketone bodies, which do feed the brain. Fasting, therefore, is associated with ketosis, which can be smelled on the breath. The ketosis of fasting, though, which is often associated with ketogenic diets, is mild, unlike the dangerous ketoacidosis of type 1 diabetes.

Krebs, who modelled himself on his Prussian PhD supervisor, the great Otto Warburg, didn't approve of my long hair (we all had long hair in those days) and he would describe me as the department's Struwwelpeter.

———————————

22

The biochemists have been warning us for nearly a century that breakfast is dangerous

The biochemists have actually been warning us for nearly a century that breakfast is dangerous, though unfortunately they did not express it like that. Back in 1921 and 1922,* two different papers appeared in German research journals describing the 'second meal' phenomenon, by which the second meal of the day is safer than the first.[1] What does this mean?

Well, the first meal of the day is the meal you eat when you break a fast, and the second meal is the meal you eat in the hours after the first meal but before you enter another fast. So if you eat three meals a day, with breakfast at 7.00 a.m., lunch at 1.00 p.m., and dinner at 7.00 p.m., then breakfast is your first meal, and lunch your second (and dinner your third). But if you do as I do, and eat only two meals a day, namely lunch at 1.00 p.m. and dinner at 7.00 p.m., then lunch is my first meal and dinner my second.

In the 1920s papers, two German researchers showed that the second meal of the day is safer than the first: i.e. for the

---

* The year 1921 is venerable in biochemistry. The world's first professorship of biochemistry was not established until 1902, in Liverpool, UK, so these early biochemical descriptions of the second meal phenomenon date back almost to the origins of the discipline.

same glucose intake, the rises in blood glucose levels after a second meal are lower than after the first (or, to express this differently, the rises in blood glucose levels after a first meal are higher than after the second). The German researchers described their findings as the 'second meal phenomenon', because they were struck by the increased glucose-sensitivity of the second meal, but the student of breakfast could call it the 'first meal phenomenon' because they would be struck by the increased glucose-resistance of the first meal. A compromiser might call it the 'first/second meal' phenomenon.

Note that this phenomenon is *not* about the circadian rhythm. Obviously breakfast is generally the first meal of the day, but my first meal is lunch, yet it would respond to glucose like a first, not second, meal. Why? Not because of cortisol (whose morning peak will have long gone) but because of free fatty acids which, of course, induce glucose- and insulin-resistance.

But when lunch is eaten as a second meal, i.e. after a breakfast, then – because of the insulin that is released on eating breakfast – the pre-lunch levels of free fatty acids are low, so the post-lunch levels of glucose are consequently also low. The first/second meal phenomenon is found in the healthy and in type 2 diabetics alike.[2]

For nearly a century, therefore, the biochemists have warned that the first meal of the day is dangerous, and since 99 times out of 100 that first meal is breakfast, they have also shown that breakfast is a dangerous meal.

PART NINE

Skipping Breakfast: Personal Stories

Here I recount what happened to me and some other people when we skipped breakfast.

23

My story, episode 2

After I realised, using my glucometer, that breakfast was bad for me, I resolved to skip it. This was a surprisingly lonely decision because in those days, back in 2010, breakfast was universally supposed to be a good thing, particularly for diabetics. Moreover, I didn't find it an easy step because I'd always liked breakfast, so initially I felt hungry in the mornings. I also felt weak. But I soon learned to cope with the hunger and weakness by adopting two strategies.

First, on waking I resort to a long strong cup of black coffee; and second I go for a run or a swim or a cycle ride. Consequently I go to work feeling fine, and I actually find my mornings more energised post-coffee post-exercise than if I'd breakfasted: the exercise pre-empts any feelings of weakness.

The exercise also obviates my hunger. A number of studies have confirmed that exercise first thing in the morning reduces hunger,[1] and though those studies also tend to show that, for most people, the hunger will return mid-morning, I find that once at work I'm so engrossed that my appetite is kept away by another long strong mid-morning cup of coffee: having exercised and coffeed, I find it easy not to eat before lunch.

Since the kitchen is never far away, and since domestic life is rarely as engrossing as work, I find weekends a greater challenge, yet the opportunities for exercise are also greater at weekends (small children and other obligations permitting) and the rule of 'not a calorie before 12.00' seems to see me through.

And not only has my glucometer been pleased by my

breakfast skipping but so has my waistline. Without even trying to slim, I've found breakfast skipping to be a sure-fire way of losing weight and of keeping it down.

Perhaps more interesting, though, than my learning how to skip breakfast as a challenge, are the experiences of the many people for whom skipping has been a liberation. Consider three people I know, DR, AM and GS.

DR is a 50-year-old male publisher who, eighteen months before I interviewed him, weighed 220 pounds (15 stones 10 pounds; 100 kg) and measured 2 metres in height (6 feet 7 inches). He thus had a BMI of 25, which – though just within the normal range – worried him because he had a pot belly. Moreover, he generally felt lethargic. He ate breakfasts daily (sometimes cereals, sometimes toast or muffins, sometimes something cooked; eaten either at home or – in the case of bacon or sausage butties – bought on the way to work) but, unhappy with his lethargy, he experimented by skipping breakfast, whereupon he made a great discovery: by skipping breakfast he liberated himself from a dependence on food. In his breakfast years he had felt 'tethered' to food, as he had once felt tethered to cigarettes, so he'd *needed* elevenses of muffins or other carbohydrates, and in the afternoons he'd *needed* similar sugar binges. He was, in his own words, on a 'rollercoaster' of carbohydrate- and food-dependence.

As Robert Crampton had described, breakfast – far from guarding against grazing later in the morning – had acted as a trigger on DR to carry on eating. His 8.00 a.m. bowl of porridge had led to the 11.00 a.m. muffin *and* to the 3.00 p.m. Victoria sponge cake. Breakfast had served to get him into a scoffin' kinda mood.

But after DR gave up breakfast those cravings left him, and he ceased to need to eat anything before lunch, nor did he need carbohydrate binges in the afternoon. Now that he skips breakfast, he has brought lunch forward by half an hour, from 12.30 to 12.00 noon, but otherwise he is less hungry in the mornings and afternoons. Moreover he now spontaneously makes healthier food choices at lunch and dinner (freed of his carbohydrate tether, he eats more vegetables) and – without having taken a conscious decision to eat less – he has nonetheless lost weight, and he now weighs 180 pounds (12 stones 12 pounds or 81.6 kg). He also feels calmer in himself – yet more energetic.

AM has a similar story. He is a 48-year-old male writer, and though he has always enjoyed breakfast, he has long been aware that if – for whatever reason – he's had to skip it, he experiences nothing untoward. In other words, after skipping breakfast, he doesn't feel unusually hungry in the mornings, though he probably brings lunch forward by about half an hour.

About five years ago, on recognising he was overweight (his waist size had risen to 36 inches) he decided – as it was an easy strategy for him – to slim by skipping breakfast. It worked happily, and over the next nine or so months he lost about 2 stone (12.7 kg). Over those nine months he noticed only one unusual phenomenon, namely that as long as he didn't eat in the mornings his appetite was unremarkable, but if at elevenses he ate a biscuit, say, a raging hunger would be unleashed and he then craved more food. So of course he abstained from eating until lunchtime.

AM would have made breakfast skipping his daily routine but for pressure from his wife and mother, who told him he was damaging his health because – as everybody knows – breakfast is the most important meal of the day and he should be eating it like a king. So he has taken it up again, generally eating granola or muesli. His weight, too, has gradually gone back up, and he now wears 36-inch waist trousers again, though they are (for now) less tight than before.

GS is a 26-year-old female economist who happened to hear from me that breakfast is a dangerous meal. GS has always been health-conscious (she usually eats salads for lunch) so she decided to skip breakfast as an experiment. Embarking on the experiment worried her because she also understood breakfast to be the most important meal of the day that she should be eating like a king (queen) so she feared she might be left cripplingly weak or hungry by mid-morning. For her first experimental day I advised her to store two large triple-chocolate muffins in her desk, to be consumed in the unlikely event of an energy emergency, but the muffins went uneaten: instead she found over the next few days that she became *less* hungry in the mornings, and she soon started to delay lunch until about 1.30–2.00 p.m.

GS also felt less hungry in the afternoons, so she now skips her erstwhile p.m. snacks (of nuts or Greek yoghurt or hummus and carrots). Even better, she feels more alert in the afternoons, and her productivity has increased. And as good, without making any effort, she found in the early weeks of her new regime that she lost about a pound of weight a week before stabilising to a new weight of several pounds lighter.

Food cravings: Like Robert Crampton, DR, AM and GS were suffering from 'food cravings'. A Canadian study on 1,000 college students revealed that two-thirds of men and almost all women (97 per cent) suffer from them.[2] They can strike several times a week, and – this is one key to understanding why breakfast makes us fat – they are generally aggravated *not* by fasting but by *eating*, especially carbohydrates.[3] Although the mechanism has not been fully characterised, we know that blood glucose levels rise and then fall following the ingestion of carbohydrates; and we further know that as those levels fall, so the levels of a hormone called ghrelin rise.[4]

Ghrelin is the hunger hormone, and its blood levels rise and fall in opposite directions from insulin's: so when our stomachs are empty or our blood sugar levels are low, the ghrelin's blood levels rise, to make us hungry; but when we eat they fall, and thus induce satiety.

Professor Christiansen showed that breakfast eaters' blood glucose levels are unusually volatile, thus precipitating an unusual number of blood sugar spikes and troughs, which will stimulate the release of ghrelin; and indeed Dr Betts has shown that levels of ghrelin are higher in the afternoon when breakfast is eaten (i.e. lower in the afternoon when breakfast is skipped) which could easily power an attack of craving.[5] So DR, AM and GS were getting their cravings because they'd eaten in the mornings, but when they skipped breakfast and morning snacks, they lost those cravings. And lost weight. And lost their lethargy.

Lethargy: One problem many people develop on eating breakfast is sleepiness or lethargy in the mornings or afternoons. DR was a morning victim, GS an afternoon victim. Actually, eating any meal – particularly a high-fat meal – will induce sleepiness, and though the mechanisms are obscure (contrary to myth, they do not involve the diversion of blood from the brain to the gut but, rather, seem to be mediated by various amino acids, hormones and nerves)[6] the phenomenon is undoubtedly real. Post-prandial sleepiness is, of course, nature's way of telling us that we're meant to eat primarily at dinner time, as DR and GS discovered when, by skipping breakfast, their daytime lethargy was alleviated.

Post-prandial sleepiness is, moreover, aggravated by diabesity, which is why Diabetes UK reports 'tiredness – particularly after meals' to be a feature of the metabolic syndrome,[7] and which is also why, in another unexpected side effect, weight loss (bariatric operations) will generally cure the daytime lethargy of the obese. So when, on skipping breakfast, DR also reversed his diabesity, he landed a double whammy on daytime sleepiness.

Nature did try to warn DR, AM and GS: in 2013 Dr Frank Scheer and his colleagues from Harvard (a different division from the nutrition people) published a study on twelve healthy young people, showing that their hunger and appetite are at their lowest level (and nausea at its highest level) first thing in the morning, while the converse is true twelve hours later, with hunger and appetite being at their highest level (and nausea at its lowest level) at dinner time, which is why people spontaneously eat less in the mornings than in the evenings.[8] In particular, Scheer found, our appetite for 'sweet, salty, and starchy foods, meal/poultry and fruits' is much stronger in the evenings, suggesting that our 'desire for high energy foods' is to eat them at dinner. Our bodies, in short, are telling us that breakfast is a dangerous meal and dinner a safe one.

Breakfast-dependency: Most people find that, after a day or two of adjusting to it, they can skip breakfast easily. In Professor Christiansen's words, of the thirteen patients he asked to skip breakfast, 'none . . . felt hungry during the mornings with fasting.'[9] In the words of David Zinczenko, who is the editor-in-chief of *Men's Health* and a skipping proselytiser, 'Your first day skipping breakfast may be difficult . . . By the end of the first month, most testers said skipping breakfast became a painless routine.'[10]

But there are those who claim that they can't adapt to skipping and that they *need* breakfast if they are to fuel their mornings. These people say they feel weak, or intolerably hungry, without breakfast. How do I respond to them?

First, I believe them. James Betts of the University of Bath Breakfast Project has shown that eating breakfast stimulates an increase in spontaneous casual exercise (fidgeting, taking stairs rather than lifts, etc.) which seems to be a subconscious response to breakfast.[11] Because the energy burned off by that exercise matches the energy ingested, that post-breakfast exercise seems to be nature's way of trying to protect us from diabesity by burning off the breakfast calories, but nonetheless people who feel weak or hungry on skipping breakfast may be dependent on that unconscious sense of energy.[12]

But what if you're breakfast-dependent but can't find an effective breakfast-avoiding strategy? What to do? I discuss this later.

PART TEN

How Insulin Kills Us

Breakfast is not only dangerous because
it is a morning meal, it is further dangerous
because it is usually a carbohydrate fest.
Carbohydrates wreak their damage by
inducing the metabolic syndrome,
which I describe here.

24

What a modern plague looks like: the metabolic syndrome

It was in 1988 that Dr Gerald Reaven, an endocrinologist at Stanford University, California, delivered his famous lecture, 'Role of insulin resistance in human disease', whose published version has been cited over 13,600 times.[1] In his lecture Reaven showed that insulin-resistance was the cause not only of diabetes, prediabetes and obesity, but also of a number of other serious disorders – including hypertension and dangerous blood fats – that tend to cluster within the same people. He described his constellation of disorders as 'syndrome X' because he couldn't think of a better name,* though we now call it the metabolic syndrome. The disorders of the syndrome include:

- insulin-resistance (leading to prediabetes and/or type 2 diabetes)
- abdominal obesity
  – for men – waist circumference greater than 40 inches (102 cm)
  – for women – waist circumference greater than 35 inches (88 cm)
- hypertension: blood pressure greater than 130/85 mm Hg

---

* F.B. Kraemer and H.N. Ginsberg (2014) have written a charming profile of Gerald Reaven, the man and his research, in *Diabetes Care* 37: 1178–81.

- HDL cholesterol
  - – for men – less than 1 mmol/l (40 mg/dl)
  - – for women – less than 1.3 mmol/l (50 mg/dl)
- triglycerides greater than 1.7 mmol/l (150 mg/dl)
- an inflammatory state
- a pro-blood-clotting state.

Not everyone with the syndrome will express all the disorders, but nonetheless those disorders tend to go together in patients.

Incidence: No one should underestimate the incidence of metabolic syndrome. We really are – to employ a cliché – discussing an epidemic or pandemic, made all the more dangerous for it being largely hidden. Reaven himself described his syndrome as a 'silent killer'.[2]

Because the syndrome is so multifaceted, doctors differ over its precise definitions, but if we apply the criteria of the International Diabetes Federation (IDF) then 40 per cent of white Americans have it. But look at the age distribution: below 40 years of age only 30 per cent of white Americans have it, but aged 40–59 the figure rises to 44 per cent, and over 60 the figure rises to 59 per cent.[3] Those are 2005 figures, and the incidence is ever rising: and since most people reading this will live to be older than 60, we can say that most white people (perhaps two-thirds of white Americans) will eventually suffer from – and will have a high chance of dying from – the metabolic syndrome. Some ethnic groups do even worse: in 2005, 75 per cent of Mexican-Americans aged over 60 suffered from it. But some groups do better: in 2005 only 55 per cent of African-Americans aged over 60 suffered from it.

Let us look at the syndrome's individual elements.

Insulin-resistance: Insulin-resistance lies at the root of the syndrome.[4]

Abdominal obesity: Some authorities place this at the heart of the syndrome. In the words of one review: 'The defining characteristic of this disease is increased visceral adipose tissue mass.'[5]

But since abdominal obesity correlates so well with insulin-resistance (hence the coining of the term 'diabesity') there is surely no need to debate which pathology, prediabetes or abdominal obesity, is the more central. They come together.[6]

Hypertension: This condition is now epidemic: some 30 to 45 per cent of Europeans suffer from it,[7] as does a similar proportion of Americans.[8]

Some 90–95 per cent of cases are of so-called 'essential' hypertension. This is not a very informative name but it means that there appears to be no obvious cause for it. Some 5–10 per cent of cases are secondary to renal or other diseases, but in essential hypertension the disease seems to have emerged from nowhere.

Nowhere? Actually, we do know what either causes it or what, at any rate, is closely associated with the cause: insulin-resistance. Patients with essential hypertension have high levels of insulin, and there is a direct correlation between plasma insulin levels and blood pressure.[9] So insulin-resistance seems to be the cause of essential hypertension, and it appears that insulin itself normally dilates blood vessels (and thus lowers blood pressure) which is an effect it mediates via a chemical called nitric oxide. That mediation, however, is impaired by insulin-resistance.[10]

As I've reported above, insulin-resistance leading to the diversion of excess energy into fat stores, makes – in moderation – evolutionary sense, but I cannot think of an evolutionary advantage for hypertension which, by promoting cardiovascular disease, kills and maims, so it was with some excitement that I recently started to read a paper with the title: 'Link between insulin resistance and hypertension: what is the evidence from evolutionary biology?'.[11]

It opened well: 'Insulin resistance has gained a bad name and is perceived as deleterious . . . however in human evolutionary history, insulin resistance may be an essential part of normal homeostatis to facilitate redirection of nutrients to pivotal organs.'

Yet though the authors of this paper really tried, they couldn't in the end find any evolutionary advantage in insulin-resistance-generated hypertension, so its emergence remains a mystery.

Perhaps the link is with obesity. Adipose tissue elaborates a chemical called angiotensin II,[12] which raises blood pressure by constricting blood vessels except, apparently, in the adipose tissue itself.[13] Curiously, adipose tissue is poorly supplied with blood and oxygen,[14] so perhaps it secretes angiotensin II to raise blood pressure to push more blood into itself. We need more research.

Cholesterol and triglycerides: There are many types of fat in the body, but here I am going to focus on two key ones, cholesterol and triglyceride.

Cholesterol: A lump of cholesterol looks and feels a bit like a lump of wax, but boring though a lump of it may appear, nobody today needs be told it is potentially a dangerous chemical. Yet it is also an essential one: it is a building block of cell membranes and other crucial structures, and if our bodies were suddenly to be rendered cholesterol-free, we would collapse into a jelly. We need cholesterol and it is, therefore, dangerous only in excess.

Because atherosclerotic lesions are full of cholesterol, it seemed obvious in the early 1950s, when atherosclerosis was becoming recognised as epidemic,[15] to suppose that raised blood levels of circulating cholesterol caused it, and a famous Framingham study showed in 1961 that raised levels of total circulating blood cholesterol are indeed associated with higher rates of heart disease.[16] But subsequent studies have failed to find such tight correlations between blood levels of total cholesterol and heart disease, so the focus of research has moved away from total cholesterol to its subtypes, including HDL cholesterol and LDL cholesterol. What are these?

Well, one problem with cholesterol, as with all fats, lies in its passage through the bloodstream. I described above how, in the guts, fats are broken into fatty acids and cholesterol, which is where the logistical problems arise. How do these fats travel through the bloodstream to the rest of the body? Sugars and amino acids are water-soluble, so they just dissolve into the blood, but cholesterol and fatty acids are oily.

To circumvent its water-phobia, a fat like cholesterol travels through the bloodstream in association with specialised proteins called lipoproteins (the words 'oil', 'fat' and 'lipid' can be used interchangeably in biochemistry, so 'lipoproteins' could have been called 'oilyproteins' or 'fattyproteins'). These lipoproteins are specialised detergents that dissolve particular fats in water.

FIGURE 24.1
A lipoprotein

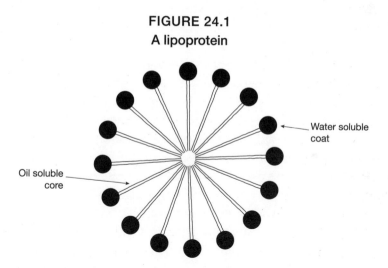

The surface of a lipoprotein is coated in proteins and other chemicals that are water soluble, while the core contains the fats or oily parts that are protected from the water.

Lipoprotein molecules and fat molecules then fuse into particles called lipoprotein particles. There are at least two types of lipoprotein particle relevant to cholesterol, namely high density lipoproteins (HDL) and low density lipoproteins (LDL). There is little mystery to these particles' names: when blood is centrifuged in the laboratory, the high density lipoproteins fall

towards the bottom of the tubes but the low density lipoproteins are reluctant to be centrifuged, and they migrate towards
the top of the tubes. The difference in the particles' density
comes partly from their different fat cores but also from their
different protein coats. In biology, their different densities per
se have no significance (the body lacks centrifuges) so we use
the different densities only as a laboratory tool.

These lipoproteins' functions are reasonably well understood:
LDLs transport cholesterol from the liver to the tissues, while
HDLs return excess cholesterol back to the liver. Consequently,
it has become fashionable to describe LDL cholesterol as 'bad'
(because it transports the cholesterol to the arteries) and HDL
cholesterol as 'good' (because it returns the cholesterol from the
arteries to the liver). Roughly three-quarters of total circulating
blood cholesterol is LDL cholesterol, while HDL cholesterol
makes up only about a quarter, and the cardiovascular risk rises
when the LDL/HDL ratio rises much above 3:1 or so.

High levels of circulating cholesterol are epidemic in the
west. In 2011, for example, the Centers for Disease Control
and Prevention reported that 71 million American adults (33.5
per cent) had raised levels of LDL cholesterol.[17] Not all surveys produce the same findings: there has been a vast public
health programme over the last few decades, and there is universal agreement that, thanks to screening and medicines, LDL
cholesterol levels within the population are falling; nonetheless,
a study from the Centers for Disease Control and Prevention
reported that most patients who are at risk from atherosclerosis
(patients with coronary heart disease or diabetes) have raised
levels.[18]

But LDL cholesterol is not the full story. We know the metabolic syndrome is the major cause of heart attacks and strokes,
but – curiously – that syndrome does *not* raise total cholesterol
or LDL cholesterol levels in the blood. Rather, it's saturated
fat in the diet that raises total and LDL cholesterol,[19] though
in ways that seem to be cardiac neutral. However, the metabolic syndrome raises the wrong *types* of LDL cholesterol: LDL
comes in different forms, including small and oxidised forms,

and those are the ones that are raised in the metabolic syndrome and those are the ones that precipitate atherosclerosis. So:

- saturated fat in the diet raises total LDL cholesterol levels (but these are apparently cardiac neutral)
- the metabolic syndrome raises the wrong types of LDL cholesterol, and these are damaging
- further, HDL levels fall in the metabolic syndrome, which will encourage cholesterol to accumulate in peripheral tissues including arteries.

Triglycerides: A lump of triglyceride looks and feels a bit like butter, because butter is indeed largely triglyceride (80 per cent). The other 20 per cent of butter is water. The fat in meat is also largely triglyceride, though of course meat also contains a range of other fats.

Like cholesterol, triglyceride is present in high concentrations in atherosclerotic lesions, but the killer triglycerides seem not to be the ones we absorb after food but, rather, the ones the liver makes. Those are transported from the liver to peripheral tissues in lipoproteins called very low density lipoproteins (VLDLs), and insulin-resistance causes the liver to make too many of them.[20]

Moreover, Jeff Volek (one of the authors of the 2010 book *New Atkins for a New You*) has found that saturated fats in the diet didn't seem to produce saturated fats in the plasma. In other words, it doesn't matter what fats you eat, they do not alter your pattern of circulating blood fats. But the more carbohydrate you eat, the more palmitoleic acid circulates in your bloodstream, and palmitoleic acid is associated with insulin-resistance, cardiovascular disease and cancer. Which means that fats in our diet seem not to damage us, but that carbohydrates are turned by our livers into fats, including palmitoleic acid, that do kill us.[21]

Being caused by insulin-resistance, the dangerous lipid changes of the metabolic syndrome are seen in prediabetes as well as in type 2 diabetes: a 1990 study from Texas on forty-three prediabetics showed they had unhealthy blood lipids,[22] while a 2002 Harvard study on nearly 6,000 middle-aged female nurses with prediabetes showed that they were nearly four times more likely than healthy people to develop a heart attack, and three times more likely to develop a stroke.[23]

Inflammation and pro-clotting: Little I've written immediately above will have come as a surprise to the average well-informed person – we all know that obesity, cholesterol and hypertension are bad for us – but people may be surprised by the emergence of inflammation and blood clotting as dangers caused by over-eating.

An inflammatory state: One of the greatest insights in recent decades has been the appreciation that inflammation (from the Latin *inflammo* 'I ignite; I set alight') lies at the heart of many diseases, including not just insulin-resistance and atherosclerosis but also cancer and perhaps Alzheimer's disease.

The Roman scholar Celsus (*c.* AD/CE 1–50) described inflammation as the fourfold response (pain, heat, redness and swelling) the body makes when a tissue is damaged. A fifth response (loss of function) was later added to the list. Three of these five responses arise because, when cells die from trauma, infection or other extraneous causes, local immune cells are activated to clear the debris, and among their actions those cells secrete chemicals that increase the local blood flow to recruit yet more immune cells from the bloodstream. The increased local blood flow will raise the local temperature (blood is warmer than the peripheral tissues, which are cooled by their exposure to the air), cause ruddiness (blood is red) and promote swelling (blood fluids occupy volume). The pain and the loss of function associated with inflammation can be attributed to the original damage to the tissue.

So far so well known. But, unexpectedly, it has emerged that visceral or abdominal fat is a major inflammatory organ. It is chronically inflamed. In the metabolic syndrome, there are twice as many immune cells as fat cells in the abdominal

fat cushion.[24] (I use the terms 'immune cells' and 'inflammatory cells' interchangeably because they can morph into – and
activate – each other.) Because the immune cells are relatively
small, and the fat cells relatively vast, the adipose tissue does
not swell up threefold in response to its infiltration by immune/
inflammatory cells, but nonetheless the majority of the cells in
the abdominal fat cushion are immune cells: it is an inflammatory organ.

(Fat cells are relatively vast because they basically constitute
a vast droplet of oil around which is stretched a desperately
thin cell. To imagine a fat cell, imagine a balloon: the air in the
balloon represents the fat, while the thin rubber substance of
the balloon represents the stuff of the cell. Fat cells are 99 per
cent fat, and only 1 per cent stuff. But immune cells consist only
of stuff, so they occupy only 1 per cent of the volume of fat
cells, so an invasion of immune cells will not obviously alter the
total volume of the abdominal fat cushion. But that invasion
will hugely increase the immune/inflammatory capacities of the
visceral and abdominal fat tissues.)

Surprisingly, fat cells are part of the immune system. We
know that immune and inflammatory cells secrete chemicals
into the blood, which then recruit more immune or inflammatory cells, and it transpires that fat cells also secrete those
chemicals. Why? Nobody knows, but it appears that animals
generally do link fat tissues to immunity. In the case of insects,
for example, two researchers from the Albert Einstein College
of Medicine, New York, report that the fat body is the animals'
major immune organ: 'For insects, an organ called the fat body
mostly mediates this [immune] response.'[25]

Why, through aeons of evolution, have animal fat cells either
retained an immune function or have, within the different phyla
and subphyla, separately evolved a joint fat/immune function?*

---

* We don't know if our immunologically involved fat has descended
directly from an insect/human common ancestor, or whether our
fat cells' involvement in immunology evolved by so-called 'parallel

The best clue comes from those very rare people who are born with a mutation of leptin-deficiency. Leptin is the hormone that is secreted by fat cells to suppress appetite, and individuals who are born leptin-deficient will grow to be very fat because there is no leptin to suppress their appetite. But up to half of those leptin-deficient individuals will die in childhood, not from their obesity but because one of leptin's jobs is to stimulate the immune system, and in the absence of leptin the immune system is dysfunctional.[26]

So leptin, which is secreted by fat cells when they are engorged, not only inhibits appetite, it also stimulates the immune system and thus keeps us alive by repelling infections. Equally, starving people have low levels of leptin, and they are very vulnerable to infection because their immune systems are suppressed.

Why? Well, animals have to make trade-offs. The first call on an energetically challenged animal (and animals in the wild may be energetically challenged because food may be scarce) is immediate body maintenance: can the animal keep its heart beating *now*, and its muscles fuelled *now*? Only if an animal has energy reserves can it afford to divert them into non-immediate tasks such as immunity/inflammation: and an animal knows it can afford to divert its stored energy only when its fat bodies are full – i.e., when leptin levels are high – because leptin levels rise in proportion to the size of the fat stores.[27]

Consequently, obese people have very active immune/inflammatory systems. Which would normally be a boon: the major

---

evolution' the way many different animals (insects, birds, bats, etc.) separately learned to fly. When I was a medical student, one of our teachers, a Jungian analyst, tried to persuade us that the human duodenal ulcer was an evolutionary inheritance from a contemporary sea-living crustacean that – when threatened by a predator – sheds its stomach lining so that the predator can feast on it and thus depart replete. 'I offer you my stomach lining, oh CEO,' the Jungian suggested we were saying when we developed a duodenal ulcer, 'please now eat that and spare me.' That Jungian wasn't a good evolutionary biologist, but nonetheless there is no reason to doubt that fat tissues and immunity have been linked for aeons.

cause of death for humans until very recently, as for many animals in the wild, was infection, so an active immune/inflammatory system was a blessing. Only now, in these hygienic times when non-communicable diseases such as insulin-resistance have emerged as our major causes of death, is a stimulation of our immune/inflammatory systems a handicap, because in the absence of pathogens our immune systems are inappropriately active.

Interestingly, leptin has a mirror hormone: adiponectin. Unlike leptin, adiponectin is released by human fat tissues when they are *depleted*: blood levels are high in anorexia and low in obesity. And its roles, too, are the opposite of leptin's, as was described in the title of a recent paper: 'Adiponectin as an anti-inflammatory factor'.[28]

So, obese patients secrete, into the bloodstream, pro-inflammatory chemicals that, in the wild, would be life-savers but which, in today's hygienic civilisation, are nuisances, because not only do we not need overactive immune/inflammatory systems, but – unexpectedly – inflammatory chemicals induce insulin-resistance. Why?

Nobody knows, but our best bet is that – like cortisol inducing insulin-resistance to divert glucose to muscles during fight-or-flight – they do it to divert glucose to the immune/inflammatory systems: when the immune/inflammatory systems are activated, they will need extra energy, so if the chemicals that activate the immune systems also induce insulin-resistance in the body, they will direct glucose to the immune cells.[29] Yet the medical consequences are grim: one inflammatory chemical, for example, is called C-reactive protein (CRP), and its blood levels correlate directly with the chances of developing cardiovascular disease and type 2 diabetes.[30]

To summarise this section, therefore, it appears that the obesity of the metabolic syndrome leads to a body-wide inflammation that reinforces insulin-resistance that, in these non-infectious times, fuels the metabolic syndrome and so kills us. And we do, probably, understand the evolutionary advantages of that biology.

A pro-clotting state: Strokes and heart attacks are often precipitated by blood clots: in the presence of atherosclerosis, it is the formation of a blood clot within an artery that often precipitates the final event that blocks the artery and thus leads to damage – sometimes terminal damage – to the brain or heart. This is why the treatment for myocardial infarcts (heart attacks) may involve the infusion of a 'clot buster' such as streptokinase.

Blood clotting depends on a large number of proteins but, in a series of fat cell surprises, it appears that some of them are over-synthesised in the metabolic syndrome.[31] Why? Nobody knows for sure, but rather than rehearse the speculation let me focus on the core message of this chapter. Most people will develop the metabolic syndrome as they age, it is dangerous, and it will be aggravated if they eat breakfast.

Breakfast and the metabolic syndrome: three experiments

What does breakfast do to the metabolic syndrome? To my knowledge, three relevant experiments (as opposed to observations) have been made. One, of course, was Dr Farshchi's, which we discussed above and whose subjects were anomalous. Another was performed by Professor Martine Laville of Lyon, France, who gave a cohort of healthy young men either large (700 calorie) or small (100 calorie) breakfasts, and who after two weeks found that the big breakfast eaters showed:

- much higher fasting and all-day triglyceride levels
- lower fasting and all-day HDL levels
- markedly lower rates of fat oxidation.[32]

Which suggested that eating breakfast precipitated obesity and the metabolic syndrome. In Dr Laville's words, with 'the strong inhibition of lipid oxidation during the day [on the big breakfasts] it may be assumed that body weight could increase with time'. Professor

Laville concluded: 'Our results do not support the current advice to consume more energy at breakfast.'

But when Dr Betts from Bath did a similar experiment, over six weeks, on healthy and obese people,[33] he found no metabolic differences between eating or skipping breakfast.[34]

The metabolic syndrome takes years to develop, so the Laville/Betts experiments confirm only (i) that breakfast does not obviously protect against the syndrome, and (ii) that we need to extend those experiments over months, not weeks.* In the absence of reliable experiments, therefore, we are like the astronomers who know only by observations that the earth goes round the sun. So we may know only by observations that mornings are a dangerous time to eat, but they're reliable observations.

---

* Because Professor Laville looked at breakfast eating and skipping within the same people at different times, while Dr Betts compared two different groups of people (one group eating breakfast and the other skipping it), it's possible that Professor Laville's more statistically sensitive approach detected a trend that was lost in the noise of Dr Betts's results, but only when these experiments are repeated for much longer times can we have confidence in them either way.

25

Can we reverse the metabolic syndrome?

The metabolic syndrome is grave, and it is aggravated by breakfast. But if – among other dietary strategies – we skip breakfast, can we thus prevent the development of the syndrome?

Well, if we can reverse the syndrome we can certainly prevent it, and here is what the CEO of Diabetes UK wrote in 2009 about reversing prediabetes: 'People with prediabetes often have the chance to reverse [it] . . . by up to 60 per cent simply through losing even just a moderate amount of weight, adopting a healthy, balanced diet and increasing physical activity levels.'[1]

So yes, we can reverse prediabetes (which is essentially the metabolic syndrome) which thus puts breakfast skipping in the spotlight. So let us expand on the issues raised by the Diabetes UK CEO, namely exercise, weight-loss dieting and also age.

Exercise and weight loss: The story with exercise should be simple. It consumes calories and should thus help us lose weight. The problem, though, is that exercise burns up surprisingly few calories. As Dr Susan Jebb of the Medical Research Council said, to lose weight 'you have to do an awful lot more exercise than most people realise. To burn off an extra 500 calories is typically an extra two hours of cycling. And that's about two doughnuts.'[2]

Or, as Professor Gately of the University of Leeds, UK, said: 'if you want to lose a pound of body fat, that requires you to run from Leeds to Nottingham [70 miles, or some 100 km] but if you want to do it through diet, you just have to skip a meal for seven days.'[3]

Exercise burns up relatively few calories because our bodies are astonishingly efficient. The average human consumes about 2,000 calories a day, which is the amount of energy a 100-watt light bulb consumes a day. So our bodies are generally using no more energy than a 100-watt bulb, which is amazingly efficient. For all our myriad activities (including powering fantastically complex brains) we burn very little fuel.

The relative futility of exercise in weight loss was confirmed by a recent trial from the University of Copenhagen, where fifty-five people were divided into two groups, one engaging in aerobic interval training at 90 per cent peak heart rate three times a week, and the other eating a low-calorie diet of 800–1,000 calories a day. After twelve weeks the low-energy diet group lost about 10 per cent of body weight (26.6 per cent body fat mass) whereas the exercising group lost only 1.6 per cent of body weight (5.5 per cent body fat mass).[4]

A further problem is caused by formal exercise crowding out informal exercise. When monitored by accelerometers, it transpires that people who exercise formally tend to 'reward' themselves by flopping about for the rest of the day, whereas non-exercisers remain more physically active (such that they might climb stairs rather than taking lifts). A recent study on children in different schools[5] found that one set of 'children did 64 percent more PE [formal physical exercise] at . . . school. But when at home they did the reverse. Those who had had the activity during the day flopped and those who hadn't perked up, and if you added the in-school and out-of-school together you get the same.'[6]

Even worse, some people who exercise can even put *on* weight, because they not only flop about for the rest of the day, but they further 'reward' themselves for their virtuous behaviour in the gym by subsequently overeating and over-drinking.*

In fact, the best weight-loss and weight-maintenance regimes come from combining exercise with calorie-restricting diets: alone, neither is optimal, but together they potentiate each other. When Dr Krista Varady, the diet expert from the University of Illinois, Chicago, distributed obese subjects between different regimes, she found that:

- those on a weight-loss diet alone lost 3 kg on average over twelve weeks
- those on exercise alone lost only 1 kg on average over twelve weeks
- but those who did both lost 6 kg.

Moreover, their LDL and HDL blood levels (and subtype distributions) moved towards the healthy ranges.[7]

Exercise and longevity: There are two purposes to exercise: one is to lose weight but the other is to increase insulin-sensitivity, and from that latter point of view a clear story emerges: exercise is good for you, period. The sheer fact of exercise increases the number of glucose transporters expressed by muscle, the mechanism being mediated by the muscle contraction itself. And as muscle is such a huge organ, the consequence is to increase glucose uptake from the blood for somewhere between four and twenty hours after a bout of intense exercise.[8] Regular exercise, moreover, leading to a modest degree of fitness, will also increase the baseline level of muscle insulin-

---

* One vigorous exerciser who, unexpectedly, put on weight (around the abdomen) was Jamie Ramsay, who in 2014/15/16 ran the whole length of the Americas (10,276 miles, 16,538 km), averaging over a marathon a day and burning up to 6,000 calories a day, yet who told *The Times* on 16 January 2016: 'There is a little layer of fat around my middle that wasn't there before. I ate what I could find and a lot of the local food was sugary.'

sensitivity: a study on over 3,000 Americans with prediabetes showed that those who dieted and took exercise halved their chances of developing type 2.[9]

A recent epidemiological paper has confirmed those studies. To tease out the relative dangers of inactivity and obesity, a large multinational team followed some 330,000 Europeans over twelve years. The team assessed exercise levels and waistlines, and recorded every death. Extrapolating from their findings, the team concluded that of the 9.2 million deaths in Europe in 2008, 676,000 (7.5 per cent) were attributable to physical inactivity while only 337,000 (3.6 per cent) were attributable to obesity.[10] The team leader, Professor Ulf Ekelund from Oslo, told the BBC that 'the greatest risk of an early death was in those classed inactive . . . physical activity needs to be recognised as a very important public health strategy. Twenty minutes of physical activity, equivalent to a brisk walk, should be possible for most people.'[11]

Professor Ekelund appears to have vindicated the 'fat-but-fit' model of health, but Professor Peter Nordstrom from Umea University, Sweden, disagrees. Professor Nordstrom and his colleagues followed 1,300,000 18-year-old military conscripts over an average of twenty-nine years (during which 44,300 of them died), finding that: 'the risk of early death was higher in fit obese individuals than in unfit normal-weight individuals.'[12] In other words, Professor Peter Nordstrom doubts that fat-but-fit is healthy. Nonetheless, through the inevitable contradictions that arise in epidemiology, we know that exercise specifically targets the dangerous fat, which is the visceral or central gut fat: when sixteen obese people from Cleveland, Ohio, were put on a vigorous exercise regime over twelve weeks, their insulin-sensitivity rose by some 33 per cent, and though their subcutaneous fat fell by 12 per cent, their visceral fat fell by 22 per cent.[13]

Summarising the accumulated research, the Academy of Medical Royal Colleges issued a report in February 2015, *Exercise: The Miracle Cure and the Role of the Doctor in Promoting It*, which noted: 'Over 40% of adults do not reach the minimum recommended level of 30 minutes of moderately intensive exercise [cycling or fast walking, say] five times a week . . . those achieving even this minimum level of activity can reduce their risk of developing heart disease, stroke, dementia, diabetes and some cancers by at least 30%.'[14]

A miracle cure indeed.

Diet and insulin-resistance: If insulin-resistance is caused by overeating, it should be reversible by weight loss. Is it? Well, we observe low insulin-resistance in patients with anorexia nervosa; they develop a heightened sensitivity to insulin, which strongly suggests that weight loss lowers insulin-resistance.[15]

And we can also experiment: so when Professor Roy Taylor of the University of Newcastle, UK, put twenty-nine type 2 diabetics on an extreme diet of only 600–700 calories a day, within two months not only had all twenty-nine lost about 15 kg (some 2½ stones) but their biochemical signs of insulin-resistance (including fasting levels of glucose, insulin, HbA1c, LDL cholesterol and blood pressure) had reversed markedly. Weight loss reverses insulin-resistance.

Diet and type 2 diabetes: If prediabetes is reversible, what about type 2? Well, that too is reversible, as was confirmed by Roy Taylor: if patients with type 2 diabetes have retained good rates of insulin secretion (and about a third have), then on losing 15 kg over two months, their diabetes will reverse.[16] Unfortunately, those type 2s who have lost their insulin cannot get that back on losing 15 kg (though they still lose their marked insulin-resistance), so the lesson is that we need to catch these people before they develop type 2, while they're still prediabetic.

How does dieting reverse type 2? A number of complex explanations have been proffered, but fundamentally the issue is simple: dieting reverses the overeating that caused the condition in the first place.[17]

Surgery, too, shows that type 2 is reversible. By 1990 a number of weight-loss operations, so-called 'bariatric' operations from the Greek *bari* for 'weight', had been developed for the treatment of obesity, and these operations included the installation of gastric bands, the creation of gastric bypasses and sleeve gastrectomies (for details please see the reference),[18] and to everyone's surprise, some 80 per cent of obese patients who underwent the early bariatric operations but who also happened to be type 2 diabetic (and many of them, of course, did happen to be type 2) reversed their diabetes. The surprise was such that an influential paper published in 1995 was entitled 'Who would have thought it? An operation proves to be the most effective therapy for adult-onset diabetes mellitus'.[19]

For a long time people believed that type 2 diabetes was a progressive disease, but the bariatric surgeons and Professor Roy Taylor have disproved that depressing idea.

My own story: When he diagnosed me with type 2 diabetes, my doctor told me the disease was progressive and would inexorably deteriorate. He prescribed oral drugs* but, he said, I should prepare myself for their eventual failure: I'd inevitably develop type 1 diabetes and then I'd be needing regular injections of insulin.

But thanks to my glucometer I soon discovered that a breakfast-skipping low-carbohydrate diet kept my blood glucose levels down, and I now run with HbA1cs at around 46, which is indeed good news (to prevent the complications of the disease, diabetics need to keep it below 48). If my disease is progressing – and in five years it seems not to have – it will be doing so only slowly.

Yet my own doctor wasn't pleased! Indeed, he complained that only one in a hundred of his type 2s achieves what I'd achieved – namely the stabilisation of the disease with an

---

* He prescribed me gliclazide, which is the drug prescribed for type 2s who are not large, but because I worried about what it might do to my islets, I asked to switch to metformin. That story is not relevant to this book; I note it only to be comprehensive.

HbA1c below 48 – yet I'd done it by flouting every piece of advice he'd proffered: he told me to eat frequently, he told me to eat breakfast, and he told me to eat carbohydrates, and I'd done the exact opposite on all three counts. But of course my doctor was only following NICE guidelines, so I forgive him. (He also told me to avoid alcohol, and I discuss that erroneous advice later.)

Age: The Mayo Clinic of Rochester, Minnesota, is one of the world's most respected medical organisations, and this is what it wrote in 2014: 'Age. The risk of type 2 diabetes increases as you get older, especially after age 45.' But the Mayo does not think that age is in itself a risk factor: 'That's probably because people tend to exercise less, lose muscle mass and gain weight as they age.'[20]

For the Mayo Clinic, therefore, the major risk factors for type 2 diabetes are overeating and physical inactivity, and the problem of age is only one of oldie self-indulgence, not one of inexorable physiological progression.

Now, age is certainly a dominating factor in society. Thanks to advances in public health, clinical medicine and nutrition, we are all living longer. Indeed, the statistics are extraordinary: in the countries with the highest life expectancies, the average life span has grown at the rate of 2.5 years a decade (or 3 months a year or 6 hours a day) over the last 170 years; and it continues to grow at that rate, so every day you live, your life expectancy increases by six hours (and in the developing world the equivalent figure is eight hours).[21] This is obviously wonderful news. But is it slightly less wonderful news if age precipitates type 2 diabetes? Or is the Mayo Clinic right in suggesting that, in itself, it does not?

Different studies have produced different results, but rather than drag the reader through them all, I have relegated them to the reference[22] because the consensus is that age per se is not an important independent risk factor for type 2 diabetes, and that its two major causative factors are the two things we can indeed modify, namely diet and exercise. Which – as long as we can persuade old people with insulin-resistance to eat less and exercise more – is obviously encouraging.

Here let me draw attention to only one point from the reference, namely that centenarians (people aged 100+) are extremely insulin-sensitive, which confirms that insulin-resistance is not an inevitable feature of ageing and which also confirms that insulin-sensitivity is associated with longevity – and vice versa, that insulin-resistance kills.[23] Gerald Reaven has shown that about half of our bodily insulin-resistance is congenital, which we can't do anything about (so some people are luckier than others), but the other half is attributable to weight, diet and exercise, which we can do something about.[24]

To summarise, therefore, dieting and exercise can reverse the insulin-resistance that underlies the metabolic syndrome, and in some patients it can also reverse type 2 diabetes. And if they can be reversed, they can certainly be prevented. The major strategies by which to control them are exercise and diet, which puts breakfast in the spotlight because some diets are better than others. In particular, the new fasting diets are emerging as useful, and these play into breakfast's hands.

26

The New Fasting Diets

When I was diagnosed with type 2 diabetes in 2010, I was advised to eat frequently – to eat at least three meals a day plus regular snacks. Thanks to my glucometer, I soon learned to skip breakfast and to cut out the snacks. Indeed, I sometimes skip lunch too. At the time people were mocking: 'Typical Terence – everybody knows that diabetics should eat little and often!' But, unbeknown to me and to my dietary advisers, the tide of thought was changing even then. The change in thinking was captured by a dietician, Amelia Freer, in her 2015 book *Eat. Nourish. Glow*:

> When I first trained to become a nutritional therapist it was common practice to teach people to eat little and often . . . three main meals a day plus two or three small snacks in between . . . meaning we can graze throughout the day in the belief it's good for us. [But] in 2008 I went to a lecture about insulin management . . . Controversially, the lecturer suggested that humans just don't need to snack . . . Most of the nutritionists in the room – myself included – gasped slightly . . . It was one of those seminal moments in life when you realised what you believed in for so long . . . might not be true after all.[1]

As Amelia Freer went on to note: 'Our hunter/gatherer ancestors didn't have a constant supply of sandwiches, cakes and biscuits nor even fruit and nuts – sometimes food was plentiful, other times it was sparse. The body is fine with that.'

The body is fine with that. Actually, the body is more than fine with that, it is finer with it. Fasting has become positively fashionable, and one expert is Dr Krista Varady of the University of Illinois at Chicago, who has for over a decade been researching the effects of fasting on humans. I have structured some of this chapter around her work.

Today, there are three prominent dietary/fasting regimes:

- conventional weight-loss dieting
  – aka 'caloric restriction' or 'calorie restriction'

- the 5:2 diet
  – aka 'intermittent fasting'
  – alternatively the 1:1 diet

- skipping breakfast
  – alternatively the 8-hour diet
  – aka 'time-restricted' feeding.

Let's look at these in turn:

Conventional weight-loss dieting, aka 'caloric restriction' or 'calorie restriction': Dr Varady opens her popular 2014 book *The Every Other Day Diet* with these words:

> Diets don't work. You've probably read that statement dozens of times, if not hundreds. But even though 'Diets don't work' has become a truism, it's not true. The truth is that *diets don't work when you diet every day*. Diets don't work because no one can endure day after day of deprivation, cut off from the foods they love . . . Diets don't work because they're unworkable![2] [Dr Varady's italics and exclamation mark.]

It's a shame they're unworkable because calorie restriction is good for us, not just as a dieting strategy but also as a lifestyle. It was in 1935 that studies first showed that withholding calories from laboratory mice prolonged their lives: if laboratory animals are restricted to only 60–75 per cent of the calories they would otherwise eat, they can live up to 50 per cent longer than usual, and they can postpone the onset of the diseases of age including diabetes, cancer, renal disease and cataracts.[3] The epidemiologists tell us the phenomenon can also be seen in humans, and apparently the islanders of Okinawa, Japan, who eat on average 20 per cent less than their fellow Japanese, tend to live several years longer than their compatriots and to produce four to five times more centenarians than do most industrialised countries.[4]

That caloric restriction should be healthy is no surprise. For obvious reasons it markedly improves insulin-sensitivity (the less the food, the lower the insulin levels, so the greater the insulin sensitivity), which also reduces fasting glucose concentrations, and both those phenomena are associated with good health.[5] It also reduces abdominal obesity.

Caloric restriction may promote good health in other ways too. Metabolising oxygen, for example, is surprisingly dangerous, because it generates chemicals called 'free radicals' that damage DNA and other vital molecules, which in turn helps precipitate diabetes, cancer, atherosclerosis and other diseases of ageing. With caloric restriction, however, the metabolism of oxygen is reduced.[6]

Nonetheless, caloric restriction as a life-extender is not likely to become a favoured lifestyle strategy for most humans, because feeling hungry all the time is no fun. There are about 50,000 CRONies (Calorie Restrictors on Optimal Nutrition) worldwide, and they are (obviously) slim, biochemically healthy and psychologically tough – not everyone possesses their willpower – but I can't see their numbers exploding: calorie restriction as a lifestyle might be fine for supermodels at the peak of their earning power, but the rest of us have lives to lead, so people looking to lose weight or to keep it down may eschew calorie restriction for one of the new fasting diets.

(Anorexia nervosa, incidentally, is not an expression of caloric restriction as usually defined, because in caloric restriction there is no malnutrition whereas in anorexia there is.)

Cyclical fasting: Manu Chakravarthy and Frank Booth of Washington and Missouri universities argue that our bodies were designed to feast-and-famine, and that diabetes and the metabolic syndrome have become epidemic not only because we overeat, and not only because we under-exercise, but also because we no longer fast cyclically.[7] Certainly, particular human cultures have adopted fasting designedly (Christians traditionally fasted during Lent, Jews over Yom Kippur, Buddhist monks at the new and full moons, etc.), and it has been shown that under Ramadan (when for a month Muslims consume nothing during the daylight hours) blood levels of cholesterol and triglyceride fall.[8]

In the laboratory, moreover, Dr Valter Longo from the University of Southern California has shown that cyclical fasting is healthy even for yeast, which are our distant relatives: so when yeast were cycled between nutritious media and water, they lived longer and could resist toxins better. And when mice were put on a calorie-restricted diet for four days out of every fourteen, they didn't lose weight (they overate on the ten non-dieting days) but:

- they lived longer
- their blood levels of glucose and insulin fell
- their abdominal fat levels fell
- their bone density and brain neurone development increased
- they developed fewer cancers.

And when Dr Longo put nineteen healthy people on a low-calorie plant-based diet for five days a month, their levels of blood glucose fell, as did their weight and their blood levels of C-reactive protein and of insulin-like growth factor 1.[9]

Fasting, moreover, may introduce variety into a lifestyle, and so may help dieters stick to their diets. For all these reasons people are now experimenting with various cyclical fasting diets, of which there are two main types.

The 5:2 diet, aka 'intermittent fasting', alternatively the 1:1 diet: People on Dr Varady's Every Other Day or 1:1 diet eat 500 (women) or 600 (men) calories (a quarter of the guidelines) every other day (to protect their muscle mass, people do not completely fast on fasting days) but they eat freely on the alternate days.

How successful is intermittent fasting for weight loss? Dr Varady has reviewed the relevant research papers and, in terms of weight loss, intermittent fasting emerged as almost as effective as caloric restriction. Which means that, unlike mice, people don't compensate for the fasting days by gorging on the eating days (when consumption rises by only 10 per cent of normal).[10] That is obviously encouraging.

As for insulin-sensitivity: well, Dr Varady found that intermittent fasting was as good as – though no better than – caloric restriction in improving it, because under both regimes the glucose- and insulin-resistant-related benefits were directly proportionate to weight loss and to weight loss alone. But until the appropriate long-term studies are performed, we will not know if the weight loss of intermittent fasting will translate into greater longevity in humans.[11]

There are a number of varieties of intermittent fasting, and the most popular is not Dr Varady's original 1:1 but, rather, the 5:2 diet, which Michael Mosley and Mimi Spencer promoted in their 2013 book *Fast Diet*. This is a fun read that, like Dr Varady's *Every Other Day Diet*, contains lots of recipes, and which also tells us that Dr Varady is 'slim, charming and very amusing'. On the 5:2 diet people eat their 500 or 600 calories on only two days a week, eating freely for the other five days, which is obviously easier than dieting every other day, and which presumably explains its greater popularity (Beyoncé, JLo, Jennifer Aniston, Benedict Cumberbatch and the former Chancellor of the Exchequer, George Osborne, have all dieted 5:2).

Dr Varady has compared her 1:1 diet with Dr Mosley's 5:2 version, and after correcting for the different fasting days per week, the two seem equally effective, although certain individuals will lose weight only on her 1:1 diet and not on the 5:2.[12]

Skipping breakfast, alternatively the 8-hour diet, aka 'time-restricted' feeding: There is a problem, however, with intermittent fasting, and Dr Varady has reported that '20 per cent of people can't tolerate the 5:2 or Every Other Day diets, but they may tolerate skipping breakfast and late-night supper every day.'[13]

Under time-restricted feeding, people fast for part of every day. They eat freely during a time window (generally about eight hours) but for the rest of the day they fast. In practice, time-restricted feeding generally means that people skip breakfast and morning snacks, but they eat lunch, an afternoon snack, and dinner – but no late-night supper. (Among the 8-hour diet's fans are Jennifer Love Hewitt and Hugh Jackman.)

Dr Varady has reviewed the relevant research papers, finding that when humans and animals eat during a window of only a few hours every day, their blood lipid patterns improve, as does their sensitivity to insulin.

Dr Varady then compared time-restricted feeding with intermittent fasting, finding that eating during a window of only a few hours every day produces better biochemical results than her own Every Other Day diet or Michael Mosley's 5:2 diet.

What a star! Dr Varady is a champion – indeed pioneer – of intermittent fasting, yet she acknowledges that time-restricted feeding may be healthier. There's scientific integrity! Dr Varady also found that, whereas some 20 per cent of subjects drop out of intermittent (5:2 or 1:1) fasting studies, only some 10 per cent fall out of time-restricted (8-hour) feeding studies.

But why is time-restricted feeding healthier than intermittent fasting? Dr Satchidananda Panda of the Salk Institute, California, has offered an explanation. In his popular book *The 8-Hour Diet*, David Zinczenko, the editor-in-chief of *Men's Health*, introduced Dr Panda thus: 'Satchidananda Panda, PhD, [is] a diminutive, energetic man whose discoveries about the new science of intermittent fasting are at the cutting edge of losing weight ... *When we eat may be as important as what we eat* [David Zinczenko's italics].'[14]

Dr Panda's key experiment was published in 2012.[15] In it, he

gave rats access to the sort of fast food we humans like to eat
(burgers, crisps and the like) and it turns out that rats like it too.
On the junk food they got fat and they also developed insulin-
resistance, liver disease and inflammation. But when Dr Panda
gave rats access to the same food for only eight hours:

- they ate as much food
- but they didn't get fat
- nor did their biochemistry (liver disease, fats and
  inflammatory chemicals) deteriorate.

Why didn't they get fat? And why did their biochemistry not
deteriorate? Well, in his paper Dr Panda showed that eating
only eight hours a day amplified the circadian rhythm in the
liver. The what?

Two circadian rhythms: The body, it transpires, possesses at
least two circadian rhythms, which can run separately from
each other. As we know, the conventional rhythm is set by the
twenty-four-hour light/dark cycle, which regulates waking and
sleeping and jet lag. But the other – the digestive rhythm – is set
by eating, and if we change our eating times, our livers and guts
then shift their cyclical activities to a different time zone: if we
shift our eating patterns by, say, six hours one way or another,
our digestive circadian rhythm then follows suit, even though
our twenty-four-hour light/dark cycle remains unchanged. So it
can be 7.00 a.m. in our pineal gland but 1.00 p.m. in our liver.

It was in 2001 that a team from the National Science Foundation published in *Science* a paper whose title summarised its
findings: 'Entrainment of the circadian clock in the liver by feeding'.[16] Or, in the words of Professor Oren Froy of the Hebrew
University of Jerusalem, for our organs of digestion 'feeding is
dominant' over the light/dark circadian rhythm.[17]

Translated, these phrases mean that our guts have their own
circadian rhythm – one that is set by our eating patterns – which
may well be out of sync with the twenty-four-hour light/dark
cycle. So, how does this entrainment – this dominance – occur?

There is an important gene known as the *Per1* gene (as in 'periodic' gene) that helps set circadian rhythms. In the pineal gland (the gland that secretes the melatonin that helps set the circadian rhythm of most of the body) the expression of *Per1* tracks the changes in the light/dark cycle. In turn, *Per1* ensures that the secretion of melatonin does too.

Other organs that follow a circadian cycle also express the *Per1* gene, but when the pattern of eating by animals is changed, the digestive organs shift their pattern of *Per1* expression from the light/dark cycle to the feeding cycle. Rats, for example, feed at night (they are creatures of the night), but when, in the laboratory, rats are fed only for a few hours, during the *day*, their livers' *Per1* cycles shift, and within three days of the new regime their livers have shifted their digestive clock by eight hours. Their pineal *Per1* expression, though, remains unaltered in following the light/dark cycle, so the rats thus operate two circadian rhythms, the pineal one set by the light/dark cycle, and the gut circadian rhythm set by the timing of meals.*

And *Per1*, like the related *Per2* and *Per3* genes, regulates the rate at which the liver synthesises glucose.[18] In fact a range of other key metabolic pathways is also regulated by the gut's circadian rhythm,[19] and when Dr Panda looked at the expression of circadian genes such as *Per2*, he found they peaked at much higher levels when the animals ate for only eight hours a day than when the animals were allowed to feed all day. The timed eating had, therefore, given their circadian rhythms a timed 'push' the way parents time their pushes when their children are on a swing. Since *Per2* controls so much metabolism, the eight-hour animals were eating when their insulin-sensitivity was at a peak, whereas the twenty-four-hour animals were eating through higher insulin-resistance – and insulin-resistance,

---

* In the experiment, the rats continued to be active primarily at night and to sleep for most of the day, and though they woke specially to feed for a few hours during the day, the waking was not long enough to disturb their pineal light/dark-driven *Per1* expression.

of course, makes you fat. Dr Panda summarised his work in these words: 'Simply limiting food intake to 8 hours gives you all the benefits – without worrying about food intake . . . dampening of circadian rhythm and reduction of fasting time are contributing to obesity and diabetes.'[20]

Professor Oren Froy has performed a similar experiment. When he allowed mice to eat for only three hours a day, the following bad things fell:

- food consumption by 7 per cent
- weight by 5 per cent
- blood levels of triglyceride and cholesterol by about 25 and 40 per cent respectively
- levels of the pro-inflammatory chemicals Il-6 and TNF-$\propto$ by about 300 per cent.[21]

And the importance of generating high-amplitude circadian rhythms was illustrated when Professor Froy fed his mice either a high-fat diet for four hours a day or a low-fat diet over twenty-four hours.[22] Whereupon the mice consumed the same numbers of calories on both diets, but the four-hour feeding mice were less obese, had lower cholesterol levels, and had higher insulin-sensitivity than did the twenty-four-hour mice.

The four-hour feeding had amplified the animals' circadian rhythms, which will have maximised the activities of key enzymes at feeding times. So it really may be true that *when we eat may be as important as what we eat.*

Mice are only mice. What about humans? The value to humans of eating only two meals a day at the same times every day was illustrated by a recent paper from Hana Kahleova and her colleagues from Charles University, Prague, Czech Republic. An extract from the long title of her paper summarises its findings: 'Eating two larger meals a day . . . is more effective than six smaller meals . . . for patients with type 2 diabetes'.

Dr Kahleova looked at patients with type 2 diabetes who were on a weight-loss diet, finding that those who ate only two meals a day did better than those who spread the same number of calories over six meals: those eating only two meals a day reduced their:

- body weight
- liver fat
- fasting plasma glucose
- insulin levels
- glucagon levels
- insulin-sensitivity[23]

more than did those who spread the same numbers of calories over six meals.*

To conclude, therefore, the cyclical fasting diets are more effective, both in terms of weight loss and in terms of health, than simple calorie restriction, and of the fasting diets the 8-hour diet is the best. And of the 8-hour diets, the one that skips breakfast, mid-morning snacks and supper will be the best of all.

Why is eating at the height of circadian rhythms healthy?

Another way of phrasing this question would be to ask: how does insulin-resistance make us fat? The 8-hour diet shows that eating at the height of circadian rhythms is to eat at a time of maximal insulin-sensitivity, which calorie-for-calorie generates the least obesity, but why and how does insulin-sensitivity translate into slimness and vice versa? Robert Henry and his colleagues from the University

----

* Dr Kahleova restricted her two meals a day to breakfast and lunch (i.e. skipping dinner) because she supposed breakfast to be the most important meal of the day – which ironically it might have been for her patients during the experiment, since they were losing weight. To maintain their health, though, on having lost their weight those patients should then skip breakfast, not dinner.

of California, San Diego, helped answer these questions in 1993, when they published a fascinating experiment on fourteen patients with type 2 diabetes.[24]

Henry's patients were well controlled by the usual standards of the disease, yet they nonetheless expressed significantly raised levels of blood glucose, so Henry did an interesting thing: he prescribed them an intensive regime of insulin (normally, type 2s are treated only with oral drugs, with insulin being reserved for type 1s). Two things swiftly followed. First, the patients' average blood glucose levels fell to normal, but to achieve that fall, their blood insulin levels had to almost double, from 300 to 500 pmol/l.

And by six months Henry saw two intriguing consequences:

- first, his patients put on weight. Quite a lot, actually, from 93.5 to 102.2 kg over six months (3 pounds a month or 1 stone in six months). And the rise in weight was proportional to the blood levels of insulin

- but this weight was gained despite a *fall* in the patients' intake of food: at the beginning of the study Henry's patients were eating an average of 2,023 calories a day, but after six months of his insulin regime their intake had fallen by over 300 to 1,711 calories a day. So the weight gain had been achieved not by increasing the intake of food but by insulin – in the face of a decreased food intake – desperately partitioning energy into the fat stores.

The lesson from this experiment is that when you are insulin-resistant, insulin is the hormone that makes you fat. And when is insulin-resistance naturally at its highest? At breakfast time.

When we eat food in the morning, therefore, we have to secrete more insulin than normal, so we fuel obesity, which, in turn, promotes greater levels of insulin-resistance (as do the higher levels of insulin themselves), so a vicious cycle is inaugurated whereby even higher levels of insulin need to be secreted to overcome the insulin-resistance, so leading to even more obesity and even more insulin-resistance. Thus, over the years, eating breakfast will fuel prediabetes and the metabolic syndrome, with all their dangerous consequences.

(Atkins and Taubes have, famously, denied that 'a calorie is a calorie,' and that carbohydrates – by stimulating insulin release – are more fattening than fats. The Henry experiment seems to confirm that insulin is indeed the hormone that makes you fat. Biochemical experiments, however, on people either fasting or gaining weight under controlled laboratory conditions, seem to show that a calorie is indeed a calorie, and that iso-caloric (same calorie) quantities of either fat or carbohydrate produce the same slimming or fattening effects depending on whether they are being restricted or over-fed.[25] These differences only show, yet again, how uncertain is our knowledge about food and diets, but one solution to this particular paradox is that under normal (i.e. non-laboratory or free-living or everyday) circumstances, carbohydrates may indeed be fattening because, as shown on a population of 270 Americans over a two-year period, they induce more hunger cravings than do fats.[26] This is presumably because insulin spikes will provoke ghrelin-induced hunger cravings.)

———————

One meal a day?: What if we take Dr Kahleova's study to its logical end? What if we eat only one meal a day? Dr Mark Mattson and his colleagues from the National Institute on Aging, Baltimore, have done the experiment, and they produced an ambiguous result. When people are encouraged to eat as much food in one meal as they would over three, their biochemistry suffers: their insulin-resistance deteriorates. Dr Mattson did not explain why, but I think the explanation may be reasonably clear: when only one meal a day is eaten, it is eaten in the presence of a fasting-induced free fatty acid-driven insulin-resistance, but when two meals are eaten, then – thanks to the second meal phenomenon – the second meal is eaten in the presence of insulin-sensitivity. Two successive meals a day seems optimal.

Yet Dr Mattson also noted that: 'when on one meal a day, the subjects would have eaten less than on three meals a day if we had not asked them to consume the same amount of food that they normally eat on a three meal a day schedule.'[27]

So when people eat only one meal a day, they spontaneously eat less in total than if they ate more meals a day, so the benefits of eating only one meal a day may outbalance the disadvantages. Why am I so sure of that? Because Dr Mattson himself has been interviewed, both by David *8-Hour Diet* Zinczenko and by *US News and World Report*, which revealed that he 'skips breakfast every day, lunch most days, and relies on his evening meal for most of his sustenance'.[28]

Perhaps Mark Mattson is modelling himself on two British actors, Joanna Lumley and Nigel Havers, who have both publicly attributed their slimness to a one-meal-a-day regime, which they confirm is common within their profession. Yet Napoleon Bonaparte might be a more substantive model: in his 2014 biography *Napoleon the Great*, Andrew Roberts reported that, as a young man, Bonaparte 'ate only once a day, at 3.00 pm', and that even on St Helena, towards the end of his life, he ate only twice a day: he would rise at 6.00 a.m. but not eat until 10.00 a.m., taking his evening meal in the early evening.[29]

To conclude, fasting is good for you, and of all the types of fasting, skipping breakfast and late-night suppers is the healthiest.

David Zinczenko's 8-Hour Diet

Zinczenko's book is a popular version of this one. Although Zinczenco alludes to research papers, he doesn't provide references, and his is a book of inspirational declamations rather than a careful, judicious and nuanced analysis of the research findings. So the back cover reads

LOSE WEIGHT AROUND THE CLOCK!
MYTH: YOU ARE WHAT YOU EAT
FACT: YOU ARE **WHEN** YOU EAT

Zinczenko's book, moreover, is packed full of recipes and exercise workouts (there are none of either in this book). Yet though Zinczenko carries his learning lightly, he has thought through the breakfast mantras:

THE LEAST IMPORTANT MEAL OF THE DAY

Let me apologise on behalf of an entire country full of fitness gurus, diet-book authors, trendy nutritionists, weight loss clinics . . . Almost all of us have been feeding you a line of bull. And we've been feeding it to you for breakfast . . . We've all seen the 'facts': people who regularly skip breakfast are 450 percent more likely to be obese. People who eat a big breakfast 'jump-start' their metabolism and burn more calories. Except that it's not true . . .

And the good news: skip breakfast . . .

A lot of 8-Hour Dieters will elect to make lunch their breakfast meal . . . Your first day skipping breakfast may be difficult . . . By the end of the first month, most testers said skipping breakfast became a painless routine.[30]

———————————

27

Type 3 diabetes (and other consequences of the metabolic syndrome)

Insulin-resistance and the metabolic syndrome do not themselves kill, but they lead to the diseases that do, of which the three major ones are atherosclerosis, cancer and Alzheimer's disease. In this chapter I explore those three terrible diseases, but exploring these three diseases has provided two surprises. First, they have illuminated insulin's *other* role.

Insulin's other role: So far I've described insulin's role in stimulating the uptake of glucose by cells, but insulin has another role: it is also a growth factor; it stimulates certain cells to grow.[1] Which can be dangerous – indeed fatal – because these cells include cancerous, inflammatory and smooth muscle cells.

The tragedy is that, when someone has developed insulin-resistance, only insulin's stimulation of the uptake of glucose is inhibited – insulin's *other* role as a stimulator of cell proliferation is unaffected. So when levels of insulin in the blood rise to compensate for the tissues' resistance to glucose uptake, its actions as a stimulator of cell proliferation are correspondingly augmented, which can lead to atherosclerosis and cancer.[2]

The second surprise is that, after decades in which it was believed that the brain was insulin-insensitive, it is now understood that some of its uptake of glucose is indeed regulated by insulin.[3] Which means that when someone develops insulin-resistance, some of the brain's uptake of glucose may be inhibited, which may in turn promote Alzheimer's disease.

Let us now look at atherosclerosis, cancer and Alzheimer's disease.

The epidemiology of heart attacks and strokes: These diseases of the cardiovascular system are essentially consequences of atherosclerosis, which used to be popularly known as 'hardening' of the arteries but which might be better described as inflammation of the arteries. The story here is one of frustrated hope. Here is an extract from the British Heart Foundation's *Trends in Coronary Heart Disease 1961–2011*:

> In 1961, there were around 166,000 deaths from coronary heart disease (CHD) in Great Britain.
> In 2009, there were around 80,000 deaths from CHD in Great Britain.
> In 1961, more than 50% of deaths in the UK were due to cardiovascular disease (CVD).
> In 2009, 32% of deaths in the UK were due to CVD.[4]
>
> [Cardiovascular disease is the sum of coronary heart disease and strokes.]

Yet the British Heart Foundation went on to lament that 'Despite this fall, cardiovascular disease remains the biggest killer in the UK,' which it attributed in large part to the prediabetic, obesity and type 2 epidemics. The UK experience is typical of the industrialised world's, and it raises two questions: why has the incidence of cardiovascular disease fallen, and what is still keeping it high?

The fall in the incidence of heart attacks and strokes can be attributed to three major factors. First, the incidence of smoking has fallen – if humanity ever scored an own goal, it was when it discovered the pleasures of *Nicotiana tabacum*. Second, two major precipitants of the atherosclerosis of cardiovascular disease are (a) raised circulating levels of cholesterol and of its dangerous subtypes, and (b) hypertension, and these conditions are being increasingly well detected and treated. But, third, there is the phenomenon of foetal insulin-resistance, which was discovered by the late, great David Barker (1938–2013), an epidemiologist at the University of Southampton, UK.

Since 1911 all babies born in the county of Hertfordshire, UK, have been weighed at birth, and when Professor Barker recovered that data, and when he set it against the subsequent health of those babies, he discovered that the smaller the baby, the greater was that baby's risk – in adult life, even seventy years later – of developing cardiovascular disease and type 2 diabetes.[5] What an unexpected correlation! Babies can be small because, as foetuses, they are malnourished, but why should a malnourished foetus develop into an adult who is prone, decades later, to the atherosclerosis, hypertension, hyperlipidaemia and prediabetes of the metabolic syndrome?

Well, a malnourished foetus has to make a choice: which organs will it protect? Will it allow all its organs to be malnourished equally or will it protect some organs at the expense of others? It appears that a malnourished foetus chooses to protect its brain (these responses are little different from an adult's: when adult mammals are starved, most of their organs shrink, the exceptions being the brain and, in the case of male mice, the testicles).[6]

So, on being starved, the foetus will deprive its non-brain organs of nourishment, and in consequence it will grow into a short adult; and to help achieve that smallness, it will induce its muscles and other major organs to become insulin-resistant, so their glucose uptake will be suppressed, to spare it for the brain.[7] And once a foetus has developed a metabolic syndrome-type metabolism, it apparently keeps it for the rest of its life.

Insulin-resistance, the metabolic syndrome, heart attacks, strokes, type 2 diabetes and hypertension are, therefore, diseases of maternal malnutrition – of poverty – leading to foetal malnutrition, and because poverty is still so common, the top ten global causes of death (Table 27.1) are dominated by the calamities of the poor, which include diarrhoea, HIV/AIDS and road accidents, but which also include the consequences of the metabolic syndrome, namely heart disease, strokes, diabetes and hypertension. Unexpectedly perhaps, these diseases are therefore not limited to the acquired metabolic syndrome of the rich.

TABLE 27.1

The top ten causes of all deaths globally (annually)

1 Atherosclerotic heart disease (7.5 million deaths)
2 Strokes (7 million)
3 Chronic lung disease (3 million)
4 Pneumonias (3 million)
5 Lung cancer (1.5 million)
6 HIV/AIDS (1.5 million)
7 Diarrhoea (1.5 million)
8 Diabetes (1.5 million)
9 Road accidents (1.3 million)
10 Hypertension (1.1 million).

The data come from the World Health Organization (2015), *The Top 10 Causes of Death*, www.who.int/mediacentre/factsheets/fs310/en/index1.html.

These top ten causes of death accounted for over half of all deaths globally. The life expectancy across the globe today is about 67 years at birth, varying from around 46 in Swaziland to 84 in Japan. In 2012 some 56 million people died worldwide, though there were many more births, 140 million, so the global population is still growing (Population Reference Bureau *2012 World Population Data Sheet*, www.prb.org/pdf12/2012-population-data-sheet_eng.pdf).

But as the west has got richer, so the metabolic syndrome of maternal and foetal malnutrition has declined (leading to the fall in cardiovascular disease the British Heart Foundation recorded), yet, correspondingly, as over-nutrition has accelerated, so too has the rise of adult metabolic syndrome, thus keeping heart disease, strokes, hypertension and diabetes among the top ten causes of death in rich countries (see Table 27.2).

It was my great namesake, the Roman playwright Terence, who urged 'Moderation in all things', and we could do worse than follow his advice today: we need to eat enough to prevent mothers transmitting insulin-resistance to their foetuses but not so well that the mothers themselves develop adult insulin-resistance.

TABLE 27.2
The top ten causes of death among the world's richest nations
(the numbers of deaths per 100,000 population per annum)

1 Atherosclerotic heart disease (158)
2 Strokes (95)
3 Lung cancer (49)
4 Alzheimer's disease and dementia (42)
5 Chronic chest disease (31)
6 Pneumonias (31)
7 Colon and rectal cancers (27)
8 Diabetes (20)
9 Hypertensive heart disease (20)
10 Breast cancer (16).

Data come from the World Health Organization (2015), *The Top 10 Causes of Death*, www.who.int/mediacentre/factsheets/fs310/en/index1.html.

One interesting difference between the metabolic syndrome of the foetus and adult is that, in the foetus, it seems unfortunately to be retained for life, but the adult-induced metabolic syndrome of overeating can fortunately be reversed, and it can therefore also be prevented. So a recent Swedish study that tracked some 21,000 healthy men for twelve years, found that some 1,350 of them developed heart attacks; but the men who avoided five particular risk factors reduced their chances of an infarct by nearly 80 per cent.[8] Those factors were:

1 Not smoking
2 Having a waistline of less than 95 cm (37.5 inches)
3 Eating a healthy diet (as defined in the late 1990s, namely

one rich in fruits, vegetables, nuts, reduced-fat dairy products, whole grains and fish; a healthy diet today would probably prioritise full-fat dairy products and go easy on the whole grains)

4 Being physically active (walking or cycling for more than forty minutes a day and exercising for more than an hour a week)

5 Drinking moderately (10–30 g alcohol a day, which equates to up to a large glass or 250 ml of wine a day).

Similar studies on women have produced similar findings on their risks of having a heart attack.[9]

Commenting on the Swedish study, a spokesperson for the British Heart Foundation said that coronary heart disease is 'a largely preventable condition' (this is a very exciting statement, which recognises that we do not need to accept the metabolic syndrome fatalistically) but that unfortunately only 1 per cent of men demonstrated all five healthy behaviours.[10] (Readers of this book will recognise a sixth healthy behaviour, skipping breakfast, but that was not studied by the Swedes.)

Height, alcohol, sirtfoods and longevity

Height: Malnourished foetuses may produce small babies who grow into adults who are short and prone to heart disease, yet there are, separately, genes that produce short and small adults, and which also – for reasons that are not fully understood – predispose to heart disease. A Leicester UK study on 200,000 people found that every 2.5 inches (6.4 cm) of an adult's height cut their risk of coronary heart disease by 13.5 per cent: a 5-footer has a 64 per cent increased risk of heart disease over a 6-footer.[11]

But before we tall people (I'm 6 feet 2 inches) get too smug, we should recognise biology as an equal-opportunities operator: the genes for height also prime cancer. An Oxford survey of 1.3 million middle-aged women in the UK between 1996 and 2001 showed that for every 4 inches (10 cm) they grew above 5 feet, their risk of developing one of ten cancers (colon, rectal, melanoma, breast, uterus, kidney, lymphoma, non-Hodgkin lymphoma and leukaemia) grew by 16 per cent.[12]

Alcohol: Alcohol is integral to a Mediterranean diet. I described above how in 2013 Dr Hans Guldbrand and his colleagues from the department of medicine in Linkoping, Sweden, found that if type 2 diabetics skipped breakfast and, instead, bundled it into a large lunch on the Mediterranean model, their post-lunch blood glucose levels were then no higher than if they had eaten only a normal lunch. But because Dr Guldbrand also provided his subjects with wine at lunchtime, we don't know how much of the Mediterranean benefits he was seeing were attributable to the breakfast skipping or the lunchtime wine, but both probably played a beneficial part.

Sirtfoods: Calorie restriction, as we know, prolongs life, and in so doing it also induces the activities of certain genes and enzymes including those known as the sirtuins. It also transpires that chemicals such as polyphenols (in chocolate) and resveratrol (from red wine) will also activate sirtuins, so a longevity-and-health industry has arisen around foods that are rich in these chemicals.[13]

University research scientists will endorse a sirtfood diet, and they will advocate the consumption of such foods as green tea, dark chocolate, turmeric, kale, blueberries, parsley, capers, citrus fruits, apples, extra-virgin olive oil, walnuts, soy/tofu, rocket, strawberries, celery, buckwheat, medjool dates, coffee, lovage, red chicory, red onions, bird's-eye chilli and red wine,[14] but other scientists are sceptical, and they suggest that these sirtuin reports are based on wishful thinking and experimental errors.[15] I am agnostic because, frankly, the sirtfoods are generally good for us anyway, but I was intrigued to read in *The Times* for 2 January 2016 the comments of a journalist who had been detailed as a guinea pig for the diet: 'I found the key to successful calorie restriction was avoiding breakfast altogether.' It appears that her success on the sirtfood diet (she lost 2 stones in three months) owed more to her not eating before lunch than to anything else.[16]

Longevity: The factors that determine longevity are of course complex. A survey of some 850 men born in 1913 in Gothenburg, Sweden, revealed that those who were still alive 100 years later, in 2013, had mothers who had also lived a long time (i.e. those men had inherited good maternal genes) and they tended also to be financially comfortable, to avoid cigarettes, to have healthy levels of cholesterol, and to drink no more than four cups of coffee a day (i.e. those men had inhabited a good environment).[17] So the study concluded that both maternal genetics and various environmental factors determine longevity, though – encouragingly – the environmental factors were stronger than the genetic factors (encouraging, because we can do something about them).

Atherosclerosis: Gruel is a type of porridge, for which the Greek word is *athera*. *Sclerosis* means 'a hardening'. So the term atherosclerosis is applied to the hardening of the arteries by a porridge-like mass that accumulates in their walls.

What is this porridge-like mass? It's pus. We're all familiar with pus from boils, and the pus of atherosclerosis is not too dissimilar. Pus is basically an accumulation of dead and dying immune and inflammatory cells (as usual, I here use the terms 'immune cells' and 'inflammatory cells' interchangeably) mixed in with other debris such as cholesterol, triglycerides and, in the case of atherosclerosis, smooth muscle cells from the arterial wall.

What causes pus? Inflammation. When tissues are damaged, they heal via inflammation, and atherosclerosis can be seen as a sustained inflammatory response to arterial damage. So atherosclerotic lesions arise where arteries are damaged – and arteries are damaged where they branch or curve. Why? Blood flow. The inner coat of arteries is delicate, and when blood flows over it in a disturbed rather than smooth fashion, it is damaged; and because the branches and curves of arteries disturb the blood flow, those are the sites of atherosclerosis.

When a length of artery is damaged, its inflammatory and repair mechanisms are activated, and under healthy circumstances such arterial repairs can be completed seamlessly: I remember as a medical student attending the postmortem examination of a slim 43-year-old lady of Indian origin who had been a life-long vegan, and her aorta was as smooth as a baby's; but many westerners' arterial repairs are not seamless, they are often atherosclerotic. Why? There are a number of reasons:

- recruiting LDL particles to damaged tissues is an important part of the healing process (tissue repair involves cell proliferation, which in turn depends on the synthesis of new cholesterol-rich cell membranes), but if blood cholesterol levels are too high, or – perhaps more importantly – if the levels of the unhealthy LDL subtypes are too high, then too much cholesterol will be deposited in the lesion, where it will provoke further inflammation because deposited cholesterol can be biologically irritating
- a similar story can be told of triglycerides
- if blood pressure is too high, the damage of disturbed blood flow is aggravated
- if blood insulin levels are too high, the inflammatory and other cellular responses of inflammation are overstimulated.

Consequently, in the metabolic syndrome the inflammation of the arteries may – instead of disappearing once the artery is healed – become 'chronic' in the proper sense of the term, because the inflammation feeds on itself and does not go away. Atherosclerosis is, in fact, just one type of chronic inflammation (atherosclerotic lesions can look like tuberculosis lesions or like the chronic inflammation of silicone breast implants)[18] but nonetheless it's a dangerously sited chronic inflammation, which is why some two-thirds of type 2s die from heart attacks and strokes: their raised insulin is a horrific promoter of atherosclerosis.[19]

Atherosclerosis kills in a number of different ways. Either:

- the atherosclerotic porridge-like plaque can rupture the inner face of the arterial wall and thus provoke the formation of a blood clot – a clot that blocks the artery and thus kills the tissues the artery normally perfuses, or
- the arterial wall may be so weakened by the plaque that it ruptures, allowing the blood to leak or even spurt out of the arterial network, or
- the plaque might slowly occlude the artery, thus leading to the gradual killing of the tissues it normally perfuses.

The fascinating paradox of cholesterol and strokes

Sometimes high levels of LDL cholesterol are good for a person. There are two types of stroke. About 80 per cent of strokes ('ischaemic strokes') are caused by atherosclerosis plaques provoking blood to clot over them and so blocking an artery, but about 20 per cent of strokes ('haemorrhagic strokes') are caused by an artery bursting, often because it is weak yet under pressure from hypertension. And though the causes of *ischaemic* strokes are the same as the causes of heart attacks, *haemorrhagic* strokes are caused by blood levels of LDL cholesterol being too *low* for the needs of the local repair mechanisms![20] (In the topsy-turvy world of haemorrhagic strokes, they are prevented by high levels of LDL cholesterol, and are therefore aggravated by statin use.)

Equally, a British study of patients with chronic heart failure showed that the higher their circulating blood cholesterol levels, the longer they survived.[21]

These data provide fascinating reminders that cholesterol is an essential chemical. Which introduces statins. There is a huge controversy around statins, and it's a controversy outwith the purview of this book. Let me simply note that statins were developed by scientists to lower circulating levels of cholesterol, so they are useful in the treatment not only of raised levels of LDL-cholesterol but also of the dangerous LDL subtypes of the metabolic syndrome.[22] Further, and independently of their anti-cholesterol effects, statins may for unknown reasons also be anti-inflammatory, which is good news.[23]

Recent guidance from the American and British health authorities is that some half of all adults over the age of 40 should take statins;[24] as the BBC reported, 'millions more people should be put on cholesterol-lowering statin drugs.'[25] This shocking advice is based on the abnormal blood lipid patterns that so many people over 40 develop as their metabolic syndrome accelerates. I think the authorities are right in their diagnosis but wrong in their recommendations. I say this because, as John Abramson of Harvard has shown, statins carry their own risks (they promote type 2 diabetes, for example) and he argues that when statins are prescribed as a precautionary measure to people with the metabolic syndrome or with abnormalities in blood fats – but who haven't yet developed a heart attack or stroke – their overall death rates are not reduced.[26]

So it's probably best to prescribe statins to *treat* people with *known* cardiovascular problems or with well-characterised risk factors such as diabetes; but we should probably try to *prevent* cardiovascular disease not by mass polypharmacy but by carbohydrate-lowering diets, lifestyle and breakfast skipping. The human race is wealthier than ever: should we not use that wealth to foster a healthy lifestyle rather than the popping of pills?

Cancer: Cancer is a disease of uncontrolled cell proliferation, and insulin's stimulation of cell proliferation (perhaps in association with a related hormone called Insulin-like Growth Factor-1) will account for the doubling in the rates of certain cancers in type 2 diabetes.[27] Insulin also stimulates, as we noted above, the immune system, which promotes inflammation – and inflammation, by promoting cell proliferation, is also a provoker of cancer. Inflammation will, moreover, stimulate insulin-resistance, thus provoking a vicious circle of morbidity and mortality. Not surprisingly, therefore, a recent study led by Professor Hense of the University of Munster, Germany, found that prescribing insulin to patients increased their risk of cancer: 'insulin therapy . . . increased the cancer risk by about 25%.'[28]

In 2010 the American Diabetes Association and the American Cancer Society published a joint report, *Diabetes and Cancer*, which found that cancers of the liver, pancreas and endometrium occur twice as often in diabetics as in non-diabetics, and that cancers of the colon, rectum, breast and bladder also showed a greater incidence among diabetics, though not a doubling.[29] The one cancer whose incidence is lower in diabetes is prostate cancer, but obesity may nonetheless increase the risk of death from it.

Overweight and obesity, being associated with raised levels of insulin, are also cancer risk factors, and the cancers with which they are most associated are breast (in postmenopausal women), colon, rectum, endometrium, pancreas, oesophagus, kidney, gall bladder and liver.

Dementia: Alzheimer's and other dementias are becoming dismayingly common in rich countries.* The Alzheimer's Association reported in 2010 that dementia was the sixth leading cause of all deaths in the United States, and that an estimated 5.3 million Americans suffer from it.[30] Every seventy seconds someone in America develops dementia, and its incidence is growing: between 2000 and 2006 it increased by 46.1 per cent, and on current trends some 11–16 million Americans will have it by 2050. As so often in epidemiology, different studies produce different findings, and a recent Framingham study has suggested that rates of Alzheimer's may be plateauing.[31] But increasing age is its greatest known risk factor, and our societies are continuing to age, and nearly half of those older than 85 suffer from it.[32]

---

* Aloysius Alzheimer (1864–1915), who described the disease, was a Bavarian psychiatrist.

The disease imposes a dreadful burden. The human burden is heart-breaking, but consider also the economic burden: nearly 11 million family and other unpaid caregivers provided an estimated 12.5 billion hours of care in 2009 to Americans with Alzheimer's and other dementias, at a valuation of nearly $144 billion, while Medicare payments reached some $172 billion.[33] Similar trends are reported in the UK and other rich countries.

Alzheimer's disease, which is the most important cause of dementia, is produced by the progressive death of brain cells, thus leading to a progressive decline in memory and brain function. It seems to be related to type 2 diabetes and to insulin-resistance, which is why some scientists now describe it as type 3 diabetes. A recent review concluded that:

> Alzheimer's disease can be considered a brain-specific form of diabetes. Alzheimer's brains exhibit defective insulin signaling . . .
>
> Insulin receptors are widely distributed in the central nervous system, suggesting that insulin has important roles in the brain. The hippocampus, a region that is fundamentally involved in the acquisition, consolidation and recollection of new memories, presents particularly high levels of insulin receptors.[34]

It seems, therefore, that as patients became insulin-resistant due to overeating, so the resistance extends to the brain and thus damages it. In 2014 the Alzheimer's Association summarised the links between insulin-resistance and dementia:[35]

Diabetes and cognitive decline

Individuals with diabetes, especially type 2 diabetes, have a lower level of cognitive function and are at higher [twice] risk for dementia than individuals without diabetes [[36]] . . . Researchers have reported a strong correlation between Alzheimer's disease and high blood sugar levels, [[37]] which [cause] a dramatic increase in a protein toxic to cells in the brain [beta amyloid[38]]. People in the early stages of type 2 diabetes have signs of brain dysfunction [39] . . . They show high levels of insulin resistance in the brain and a reduced ability to use glucose to fuel normal brain function . . . In a study of nearly 15,000 people with type 2 diabetes who were aged 55 and older, people who started on metformin, an insulin sensitizer, had a significantly reduced risk of developing dementia.

[points in square brackets from me.]

The similarities between the insulin-resistance of type 2 diabetes and Alzheimer's disease were highlighted in a study from the National Institute of Aging in the USA which showed that a protein called Insulin Receptor Substrate 1 (IRS-1), which mediates the effects of insulin, is even more inhibited in Alzheimer's disease than in type 2 diabetes.[40]

Prevention: The mantra in the field is 'what's good for the heart is good for the brain,' and – though the epidemiological evidence has yet to prove unequivocally that a healthy lifestyle will prevent or treat the disease – the conventional advice has long been a healthy lifestyle,[41] as was reinforced by a randomised controlled trial from Finland: the Finnish researchers identified some 2,500 normal people (aged 60–77) who had the seven contributory risk factors (namely, low education, hypertension, obesity, diabetes, physical inactivity, smoking and depression), and they reported that if those seven factors were addressed aggressively, the patients' decline was reducible and perhaps even preventable.[42]

Recently, however, the mantra of 'what's good for the heart is good for the brain' was challenged by a vast study (on nearly 2 million people, average age 55, who were followed over nine years) from the London School of Hygiene and Tropical Medicine. The LSHTM researchers found that the *thinner* a person, the greater were their chances of developing dementia.[43]

It's hard to make easy sense of this unexpected result, but people with Alzheimer's lose weight, so presumably those people who had already embarked down the road to Alzheimer's had already lost weight, thus short-circuiting the findings. The latest epidemiological studies, moreover, have recapitulated the earlier ones: a recently published study on some 1,400 people in Baltimore, MD, showed that the higher the BMI at age 50, the greater were a person's chances of developing the disease.[44] And Tim Spector and his colleagues from King's College London, on studying some 300 healthy female twins, found that their leg muscle strength (an index of their physical fitness) correlated strongly with their protection from dementia and indeed with their brain size: physical fitness protects against Alzheimer's disease.[45]

To coin a cliché, we need more research, but it's good to note that after many years in which Alzheimer's research apparently floundered, it seems to have been reinvigorated. Between 2002 and 2012, over 400 drug trials were performed on Alzheimer's disease, of which 99.6 per cent failed.[46] The comparable failure rate for cancer drug trials is 81 per cent, so this new insulin-orientated thinking is welcome.

To conclude, therefore, systemic insulin-resistance will raise our chances of dying from atherosclerosis and cancer because the raised blood levels of insulin will power the stimulation of cell proliferation. Meanwhile, localised insulin-resistance will probably power Alzheimer's disease. These diseases are becoming epidemic alongside the epidemics of the metabolic syndrome and type 2 diabetes, which renders a re-evaluation of breakfast an urgent matter.

PART ELEVEN

If You Must Eat Breakfast, What Must You Eat?

Q: Some people cannot survive without their morning meal: what should they eat?

A: The ideal breakfast would probably be a boiled egg or two, followed by strawberries and cream. Let me explain why.*

---

* When Paris Hilton went to prison, she was given a surprisingly healthy breakfast of a boiled egg and an orange (www.dailymail. co.uk/tvshowbiz/article-484973/paris-loses-cool-mocked-chat-king-letterman.html). Oranges are of course fruit, but other than bananas, watermelons and grapes, fruit generally have low glycaemic indices and loads, and oranges are not unhealthy. Strawberries, though, have lower glycaemic indices and much lower glycaemic loads, so they are healthier.

28

So, what to eat?

So, if we remove carbohydrate from the diet, with what do we replace it?

Meat: The problem with meat, especially red meat, is that it seems to be pro-inflammatory. In 2009 an Iranian group reported in the *Journal of Nutrition*, which is published by the American Society for Nutrition, a study on 482 female teachers in Tehran, finding that the 20 per cent of teachers who ate the most meat were twice as likely as the bottom 20 per cent to have metabolic syndrome.[1] That was a cross-sectional survey, so those findings may be only associations (prosperous people may eat more meat, and be more sedentary, and eat too many carbohydrates and fat as well), but in 2013 – on pooling the findings from forty-six publications – a German research group reported that meat eaters tended to have high levels of CRP (the circulating blood marker of inflammation) while vegetable or fruit eaters tended to have low levels.[2] And since inflammation potentiates atherosclerosis and type 2 diabetes, it is not surprising that people on vegan diets have lower levels of LDL cholesterol[3] and lower rates of cardiovascular disease.[4] Indeed, a Washington DC study of forty-nine middle-aged type 2 diabetics who transferred to a vegan diet showed that:

- their fasting blood levels of glucose fell by 2.6 mmol/l from 9.9 to 7.1
- their circulating blood levels of triglycerides and LDL cholesterol fell as markedly

- the amount of protein in their urine (a marker of renal damage) halved.[5]

Unsurprisingly, therefore, epidemiological studies confirm that eating meat is unhealthy, and three large surveys in America and Europe on over a million people who were followed for a minimum of ten years, during which some 120,000 of them died, did indeed find that eating an extra portion of red or processed (sausages, salami, bacon) meat a day could increase the risks of dying from cardiovascular disease or cancer by 10 per cent or more.[6]

The much lower quantities of meat eaten in Asia, however, seem to be safe, so it appears that a little fresh meat is healthy but that Europeans and Americans eat, on average, at least twice as much as they should.[7] The epidemiological studies suggest, though, that poultry seems not to be dangerous. For all these reasons – and for environmental reasons – the Dutch government has taken the lead among governments in advising we eat meat only twice a week, and that most of that meat should not be red.[8]

What are red, white and dark meats: or why is poultry relatively safe?

There are, essentially, two types of muscle. White muscle specialises in sprints, whereas red muscle specialises in the longer haul. Compare chicken and duck breasts: a chicken breast is white because a chicken uses its breast muscles only briefly (when it flies up to a roost) whereas a duck will fly significant distances, so its breast meat is red (or dark, see below).

The biochemistry of these two types of meat is different. Breast meat – because it is only converting stored glycogen to lactic acid in a burst of wild activity – doesn't use much oxygen, whereas red or dark meat is in it for the duration so it oxidises fats to CO_2. Which is where the colour comes in, because that oxidation requires muscle myoglobin, which is similar to the blood's haemoglobin and which shares a similar red colour. Other coloured compounds such as cytochromes (*cyto*, 'cell'; *chrome*, 'colour') are also involved in meat's oxidation of fats, so the words 'red' and 'dark' for meat describe essentially the same thing.

It appears that white meat is safe to eat but that red/dark meat is less so. The connection between red meat and colon cancer is well-established, and it seems that red meat might be inflammatory because it contains a chemical called carnitine, which helps the oxidation of fats and which may be converted by gut bacteria into inflammatory chemicals.[9]

(The word carnitine comes from the Latin *carno* or *carnis*, meaning 'meat'. We get the word 'carnival' from the same source because meat-eating festivals such as Shrove Tuesday or Mardi Gras once preceded meat-free periods such as Lent; the derivation of the word 'carnage' is similar.)

So, which supermarket meats are red and which white? Basically, the major farmed meats (beef, lamb and pork) are red, whereas chicken breast is white. Chicken thighs, though, are dark or red. Some cuts of farmed meat are claimed to be white (and indeed might be) but claims in nutrition are so distorted by powerful lobbyists that it can be hard to determine their veracity by the meat aisle. Sadly, moreover, people do not trust government advice: according to the *Wikipedia* entry for 'Red Meat', for example, we're safer following the advice of bodies like the Harvard School of Public Health because: 'the United States Department of Agriculture (USDA) . . . has to contend with lobbying'.[10]

And the Harvard School advises us to eat only limited amounts of meat other than poultry (I think they actually mean chicken breast) because all other meat in supermarkets is, Harvard implies (their own advice is somewhat cryptic), red.[11] The Harvard School of Public Health has its own biases (breakfast not being the least of them), but on meat safety and colour it's probably our best guide: other than chicken breast, supermarket meat is probably red and therefore less safe.

Vegan?: Although excessive meat carries its risks, there seems no need to go vegan. Salmon is rich in omega 3 polyunsaturated fats, and a Dutch study has confirmed that salmon in the diet will lower blood CRP levels.[12] (Since 1971, when it was reported that Greenland Inuit had exceptionally low rates of heart disease, even though they ate almost nothing but fish and meat,[13] omega 3 polyunsaturated fats have been seen as cardioprotective.[14] In 1971 Inuit were still called Eskimos, which is a word of Native American origin meaning 'people eating raw meat'.)

Salmon is a fatty fish, and cod is lean, and cod is not rich in omega 3s, yet cod also lowers CRP levels, so fish generally seems to be good for us.[15] (This is a book on food, not an ethics soapbox, so I hope I don't appear sanctimonious when I suggest we should eat fish only sustainably. The Marine Conservation Society (MCS) is a respected British charity – Prince Charles is their patron – whose website provides useful information at www.mcsuk.org/. Other countries have similar bodies, though I fear they all, the MCS included, accept corporate support. Meanwhile, the Dutch government now recommends we eat fish only once a week, as that optimises sustainability while still yielding the cardiovascular benefits.)[16]

Other animal products, too, appear to be healthy. When a Connecticut group administered three eggs a day to a group of overweight men, by twelve weeks their CRP levels had fallen significantly.[17] Equally, a study from the University of East Finland on some 2,300 middle-aged men, followed over nineteen years, found that those men who ate four eggs a week had a 30 per cent lower risk of developing type 2 diabetes than those who ate only one or no eggs a week.[18] They also had lower levels of CRP and blood glucose. Eggs are good for us. (I hope I'm not sanctimonious to suggest that, from kindness to sentient animals, we should eat eggs only from free-range chickens, and that we should eat only medium-sized eggs, as laying large eggs may be painful.)

And we may want to eat animal products, if only because a survey from the University of Florida that pooled the findings of eighty-seven separate studies concluded that high-protein diets helped protect against the muscle loss of weight-loss diets.[19] There are of course non-animal sources of protein – and a vegan diet is an honourable diet – but safe animal products such as eggs contain vitamin B12 with which vegan diets otherwise need to be supplemented, and since we humans evolved to be omnivores, I suspect that an omnivorous diet may be a healthy diet.

(I'm not going to write any further outside my breakfast brief, but on the subject of animal ethics let me refer to the Compassion in World Farming (CiWF) website, www.ciwf.org.uk, and to the CiWF CEO's heart-breaking 2014 book *Farmageddon: The True Cost of Cheap Meat*.)[20]

Dairy?: It is emerging that full-fat dairy products are healthy. A Swedish survey of some 27,000 middle-aged people, followed over fourteen years, found that nearly 3,000 of them developed type 2 diabetes, but those who ate full-fat dairy products such as cream, milk and cheese were significantly protected[21] (though the survey confirmed that eating meat increased the chances of developing the disease). And a study from Quebec, Canada, that pooled the results of eight published papers, showed that eating dairy products had no deleterious (and might have had beneficial) effects on inflammatory markers.[22] Full-fat yoghurt and cheese appear to be healthier than butter, presumably because yoghurt and cheese are microbial-rich, and a diverse gut microbial population (see below) is associated with good health.[23]

Full-fat yoghurt and other dairy products are, moreover, healthier than their low-fat equivalents because – to maintain their palatability – low-fat products are supplemented with sugar. Since those products were formulated to appeal to health-conscious people, that is a cruel irony.

Eco-Atkins?: If, on a low-carbohydrate diet, we are also to lower our red and processed meat intakes, what can we eat instead? A Toronto research group has experimented with an 'Eco-Atkins' diet, which they so named because they followed

Atkins in substituting fats and oils for carbohydrates but they used vegetable not animal fats.[24] The researchers followed a group of middle-aged men and women who had abnormal blood lipid levels, and over six months the replacement of carbohydrates with vegetable oils (the diet was rich in nuts, soy products, avocado, fruits, vegetables and vegetable oils) led to insulin-resistance and plasma blood lipid levels adopting a significantly healthier pattern.*

Eco-Atkins and me: Although the scientific consensus is that eating certain animal products including dairy and non-red meat is safe, I – using my glucometer – have found that when I, personally, eat too much cheese or other dairy products, my morning blood glucose levels start to creep up. But if I go vegan for a few days (a very few days, two generally does it) they come down again. I assume that when fats from animals enter my cell membranes they do so in ways my body doesn't like (other people's bodies may be different), but when I replace them with plant-based fats my blood glucose control soon improves. That was a discovery I would not have made but for my glucometer.

Frying?: The dietitian Joe Leech has summarised the current state of knowledge in a friendly post on the web, and he has concluded that the optimal oils and fats for frying are different from those to eat uncooked. So polyunsaturated vegetable oils including soybean, corn, canola/rapeseed, cottonseed, sunflower and others, which have long been recognised as healthy when consumed uncooked, are to be avoided in frying because, on heating, they oxidise into dangerous compounds. Peanut oil, too, may be hazardous fried, while palm oil may be environmentally damaging. But coconut oil (very saturated) and

---

* Dr Mark Hyman, who is one of Bill Clinton's medical advisers, has popularised the Eco-Atkins as the pegan diet (*p*aleo + veg*an* = p*egan*) and his website advises us which foods are pegan (drhyman.com/com/ blob/2014/11/07/pegan-paleo-vegan/. Accessed 4 January 2016).

animal fats such as lard, dripping and ghee are fine when fried, as is clarified butter, though butter itself may contain proteins and carbohydrates that burn dangerously when heated. That old standby, olive oil (monounsaturated) is fine fried (though its flavour can go off on prolonged cooking), as is that new standby, avocado oil.[25]

And it goes without saying that trans fats are dangerous and should be avoided. Sadly, some countries have not yet banned them completely: in the USA, for example, up to 4 per cent of fat intake may be of trans fats. It should be 0, as in Denmark.

Nuts: Which nuts are best? They are probably all good for us, but walnuts, which are particularly rich in omega 3 polyunsaturated fats including linoleic acid, may be particularly healthful: a Harvard and Singapore survey of some 140,000 nurses showed that those who regularly ate walnuts enjoyed a significantly lower risk of developing type 2 diabetes, though such an observational study cannot, of course, prove cause and effect.[26]

Most nuts are rich in omega 6 polyunsaturated fats, which some researchers fear may neutralise the benefits of the walnuts' omega 3s but which other researchers find are associated with good health.[27] Many nuts moreover (like soy, beans and many vegetables) are rich in phytic acid, which may possibly inhibit the absorption of iron, calcium and other minerals. Nonetheless, epidemiological papers generally give nuts a good bill of health, so presumably – as in so many other areas of life – we should abjure extremes: eat lots of nuts but don't eat only nuts!

Fruit and fibre: Dr Lustig has confirmed that fruits, though rich in sugar, are also rich in fibre – and the benefits of the fibre seem to balance out the risks of the sugar, because the consumption of fruits seems to lower the risk of developing type 2 diabetes.[28] As Dr Lustig told *The Times* on 20 April 2015, fruit:

'comes with its inherent fibre, and fibre mitigates the negative effects. The way God made it, however much sugar is in a piece of fruit, there's an equal amount of fibre to offset it.'[29]

Fibre consists of long chains of plant-derived carbohydrates that, for various chemical reasons, we cannot digest. Some can be digested by our gut bacteria (to produce those embarrassing gases) but nonetheless much of our stools consist of fibre, which – fortunately – has resisted any form of digestion. Fortunately? Well, one advantage of fibre is that it slows the rate of uptake of glucose and fructose (it lowers the glycaemic index, see below) and so pre-empts the post-meal glucose spikes that can otherwise be dangerous. Fibre also encourages the anti-obesity bacteria to proliferate at the expense of the pro-obesity bacteria (see below) and it binds cholesterol and thus helps excrete it via the faeces. Fibre is a good thing.

The best fibre comes within the fruit and vegetables in which it grows naturally: even smoothies' fibre, having been mechanically sheared, is inferior to inherent fibre. And any fibre you add to your food, though better than nothing, is less useful than that which comes naturally within fibre-rich foods.

Fast, processed and junk foods: why are they so bad for us?: One emerging reason is bacteria. We have trillions of bacteria in our guts (mainly in the large intestine), and a Cambridge team has shown that over half of our stools are composed of bacteria.[30] We have up to 1,000 different species of faecal bacteria, and to discover what they do, scientists such as Fredrik Backhed and his colleagues from Washington University, St Louis, MO, will deliver baby mice by caesarean section, to raise them free of bacteria; and such mice grow up to be thin, thus showing that our gut bacteria digest food that we mammals – lacking certain key enzymes – cannot. As the title of Backed's paper showed – 'Mechanisms underlying the resistance to diet-induced obesity in germ-free mice' – even if such mice are fed a western-style burger-and-chips diet, they fail to get fat.[31]

But when germ-free mice are inoculated with human faeces, the human bacteria colonise their guts, and their absorption of food improves. Yet different people have different portfolios of gut microbial species, and these differences are not random:

so large people (including pregnant women, who of course eat for two) have different portfolios from slim people; and when germ-free mice are inoculated with faeces from large people, those mice tend to become positively fat and to develop insulin-resistance.[32] Thus we can see that our gut bacteria help determine our tendency to insulin-resistance and thus our weight.

In his 2015 book *The Diet Myth* Tim Spector shows how, when we eat fast, processed or junk food, our gut bacteria change from a non-obesity portfolio to an obesity one, whereas real food helps top up our healthy bacteria. Real cheese, for example, is packed full of good bacteria, which inoculate our guts healthily, whereas fast, processed and junk food is mono-tonically about meat, chips and sugary drinks, which contain few good bacteria.[33] Processed foods also tend to be emulsifier-rich, and such emulsifiers (detergents) may further damage the balance of gut bacteria.[34] No wonder Michael Pollan, the journalist who is known for his aphorism 'Eat food. Not too much. Mostly plants,'[35] also said, 'Don't eat anything your grandmother's microbes wouldn't recognise as food.'

Another reason fast, processed and junk foods are unhealthy is that they lack fibre. As Dr Lustig said: 'What is the definition of fast food? It's fibre-less food . . . [for reasons of storage] the food industry removes fibre from food.'[36]

Summary: So there we have it: avoid refined carbohydrates and avoid red (and processed) meat and avoid other processed foods and eat lots of plants and you're set. The major problem with such a diet is cost. As George Orwell described in Chapter 6 of his 1937 book *The Road to Wigan Pier*, the poor in the north of England spent:

> nothing on fruit; but they spend one and nine [pre-decimal British currency] on sugar (about eight pounds of sugar) and a shilling on tea . . . [theirs] is an appalling diet but the peculiar evil is this, that the less money you have, the less inclined you are to spend it on wholesome food . . . [when] you are harassed, bored and miserable, you don't want to eat dull

wholesome food. You want something a bit 'tasty'. There is always some cheaply pleasant thing to tempt you.

Today, though, people do not plumb the desperate poverty of 1930s Britain, and wholesome food has become cheaper. It should be affordable by most.

Conclusion: Ancel Keys lived to be 100, and he followed a Mediterranean diet, so if we do as he did and not as he said, and if we too followed a Mediterranean diet as actually followed by many of the people who live around the Mediterranean shores, then we too would:

- skip breakfast
- drink wine with our meals, in moderation
- feast on olive oil, vegetables, fruit, nuts and legumes (peas, beans, lentils, chickpeas)
- partake judiciously of fish, poultry and eggs
- eschew red meat, processed meat, cereals, potatoes, rice and bread
- condemn and damn sweet foods and drinks including cakes, jams, fruit juices, sodas and anything containing household sugar.

And, who knows, perhaps we too would live to be 100.

29

And if you must eat breakfast?

What to eat if you must eat breakfast and if you're insulin-sensitive? Here is the good news. If you're slim, fit and young, and if you can't find an effective breakfast-avoiding strategy, then there's no reason why you shouldn't eat it! As long as you avoid carbohydrates and sugar, there's no reason not to enjoy it. You're a member of a privileged minority (fit, slim and young) so you could claim the eating of a low-carbohydrate breakfast as a bonus, one you've earned by being healthful.

But to stay healthful, you'll need to be careful in your eating choices. Protein and fat will both be good for you, so eggs would make a useful morning meal. But since most morning meats and fish (bacon, sausages, kippers, smoked haddock, smoked salmon and so on) are – to render them piquant – processed or smoked, they should probably be eschewed (so in his 1669 assertion that 'Two Poched Eggs with a few fine dry-fried collops of pure Bacon, are not bad for break-fast,' Sir Kenelm Digby was only half right).

Also to be eschewed are croissants and cake and toast and jam and honey and marmalade and fruit juices – they are the foods of the devil – as are baked beans (which are packed with sugar) and almost everything that comes in a tin or packet. Breakfast cereals, meanwhile, are not just foods of the devil, they are the actual devil incarnate, sitting on your kitchen table, and they should be consigned to the eternal flames as quickly as possible, preferably unopened, via the rubbish truck on its way to a municipal incinerator. (Breakfast carbohydrates will raise the blood glucose levels even of healthy people and thus help trigger the metabolic syndrome.)

And porridge, I'm afraid, is also bad for you. People find that hard to believe (just as many Japanese people find it hard to believe that white rice is dangerous) but I'm afraid the cardiac death rates in Scotland are not just the product of whisky – porridge plays its ignoble share in that holocaust.* Muesli is another emanation from the nether regions, made even worse by its false pretence to health (look at its composition on the packet).

Yet here is some good news: berries such as strawberries and blueberries have surprisingly low glycaemic indices and loads (they have pleasantly low levels of sugar, and they come with fibre) and when served with lashings of cream (we know that dairy products are good for you) they are delicious, so they're safe (there's less sugar in cream than in full-fat yoghurt; almost all low-fat yoghurts are, of course, sugar bombs and therefore deadly).**

Glycaemic index and glycaemic load

Glycaemic index: This measures the spikes in blood glucose levels caused by different foods. By definition, glucose has a glycaemic index of 100, and most carbohydrate foods come in somewhere between 50 and 100. Some foods such as baguettes or scones

---

* The age-standardised death rates from cardiovascular disease were 78 in England in 2010/12 but 99 in Scotland (*Cardiovascular Disease Statistics 2014*, British Heart Foundation, p. 27, www.bhf.org.uk/~/media/files/research/heart-statistics/bhf_cvd-statistics-2014_web.pdf).

** To reiterate, dairy products in excess aren't so good for me, and if I eat too many of them over too long a period (a couple of weeks or so) I have to go vegan for a day or two until my morning glucose levels revert to the normal range. But that's my personal idiosyncrasy.

have GIs that are almost as high as glucose, in the 90s. Cornflakes and baked potatoes come within the 80s. The different pastas, on the other hand, which require significant digestion, have surprisingly low GIs of *circa* 40. But they have high glycaemic loads.

Glycaemic load: This reflects the total amount of carbohydrate in a food, and thus reflects their sustained pressure on the insulin system. So strawberries have, as might be expected, GIs of around 40 (their fibre content dampens their sugar effects) but because they actually contain few carbohydrates other than sugar, their glycaemic loads are low, at around 1.

The formula for calculating the GL of a portion of food is

$$GL = GI \times carbohydrates \div 100$$

so we can talk about the total GL of a meal. So 100 g of glucose would have a GL of 100 x 100 ÷ 100, i.e. 100.

A serving of food with a GL of 20 or more would be high, one of 10 or less be low, and one of 10–20 medium. Among common foods, baked potatoes have one of the highest GLs, at 26, while other forms of potato (mashed, boiled) come in the mid-teens. The pastas come in at the high teens or perhaps nudging 20. Cornflakes have high GLs (21) as do sultanas (25) and rice (22).

Ideally, food should have low GIs *and* low GLs, and Jennie Brand-Miller (whom we met earlier over the Australian/British paradoxes) has constructed two comprehensive lists of different foods and their glycaemic indices and loads. The earlier one is introduced by a useful if scholarly essay,[1] while the later one provides an even more comprehensive list of foods.[2] Harvard have supplied a useful abbreviated version for common foods.[3]

When planning your diet, and if you're insulin-resistant, and if you're therefore trying to minimise your food's GIs and GLs, my advice is to eat to your glucometer, because everybody's metabolism is different, but Brand-Miller's tables can provide a useful pointer.

———————

Cheese, as in a typical breakfast from the Netherlands, makes a good breakfast choice; and it's better to go for real, unpasteurised cheeses rather than the processed types (unless of course you're pregnant or have some other reason to avoid real cheeses) but you should eat them on a lettuce leaf, not on bread or a biscuit. Waffles from Holland's neighbour in Belgium, though, are out, as are the sweet liquids (maple syrup, chocolate sauce etc.) that people pour over them. Butter's probably OK, but since you won't be eating bread or toast or biscuits, you won't be needing that unless you've put it in your scrambled eggs. Margarine should be avoided as it contains processed fats.

So if you have to eat breakfast, I recommend eggs (cooked any style as long as you use only butter) followed by strawberries and cream. And if you're really hungry, cheese on lettuce should finish things off nicely.

Breakfast-dependent but insulin-resistant: Here, I'm afraid, the story is severe. Breakfast will kill you. Under no circumstances should you eat it. Insulin-resistance is a deadly condition that you must must *must* reverse, and skipping breakfast is the first step back to health; the second step being to adopt a low-carbohydrate diet.

Who is insulin-resistant?: In an ideal world we'd measure insulin directly in people, and thus diagnose them as insulin-resistant before they'd progressed to prediabetes, but that is a luxury most of us are denied. Yet it is easy to diagnose prediabetes (by HbA1c, fasting blood glucose levels or a glucose tolerance test) and that is so undertreated that we should not let the best be the enemy of the good and we should start to treat that properly. So, who's at risk of prediabetes? Whom should we screen?

Well, our sixteenth-century guides weren't far wrong when they advised us that 'two meals a day are adequate for a rest man,' and to 'eat three meals a day until you come to the age of 40 years,' and to 'feed only twice a day when you are at man's age,' because according to the American Diabetic Association, the people who are at risk of prediabetes are adults who are overweight (BMI greater than 25; greater than 23 if Asians) who additionally are:

- over 45 years old
- inactive physically.[4]

Moreover, adults who:

- have first-degree relatives with diabetes
- or are members of African, Latin, Asian among other ethnic groups, are also at risk.

While people who have:

- raised blood pressure
- cardiovascular disease
- abnormal cholesterol levels, including a high-density lipoprotein (HDL) cholesterol below 0.9 mmol/l or a triglyceride level above 2.82 mmol/l
- a history of gestational diabetes or have given birth to a baby who weighed more than 9 pounds (4.1 kg)
- a history of polycystic ovary syndrome
- any other condition associated with insulin-resistance have almost certainly already developed the metabolic syndrome.

According to the ADA, everyone who fulfils any of these criteria should be screened for prediabetes every three years. And if they're diagnosed, then:

- breakfast skipping
- low-carbohydrate diets
- exercise

should obviously provide the cores of their therapy. Yet I'd argue that everyone on the ADA at-risk list should – even if they're not yet prediabetic – skip breakfast: they're all at risk of insulin-resistance, and one way of obviating that risk would be to skip.

Their other necessary step would be to adopt a low-carbohydrate diet. There is no formal definition of this, but the American Academy of Family Physicians classifies such a diet as one that provides less than 20 per cent of calories as carbohydrates (20–60 g a day). There are a number of popular diets (Zone Diet, Carbohydrate Addict's Diet, the later phases of the South Beach Diet, the Atkins Diet etc.) that detail such a regime, and in general they involve skipping sweets, candies, baked goods, bread, potatoes and other starchy vegetables, rice, cereals and sweet and starchy fruit, but they do not preclude eating vegetables and fruit with low glycaemic indices and loads.[5]

What if you're insulin-resistant and you still insist on eating breakfast?: Well, there are people who still smoke. Ultimately your fate is in your own hands. Just as smokers trade their life expectancies against the pleasures of tobacco, so you too have to decide where your priorities lie, but if you are going to indulge, please minimise the risks by eating absolutely no sugar or processed carbohydrates.

The only exceptions to this injunction can be airline pilots, heart surgeons and other professionals who bear responsibility for other people's lives. Professionals owe their clients their peak performance, so they must eat what works best for their performance even if that includes refined carbohydrates or sugar; but let them (as they are lowered into their premature graves) remember that no one will thank them for shortening their own lives for the sake of their clients'.

Breakfast and type 2 diabetes: The dangers of prediabetes are, of course, mediated by the raised insulin levels, but the dangers of diabetes itself are further aggravated by the raised levels of glucose, and Professor Roy Taylor has found a way of obviating those.

Some 2,500 years ago Hippocrates, the Father of Medicine, said the most important part of a doctor's work was diagnosis, because without a diagnosis there can be no prognosis and no treatment. Well, Professor Taylor is a rare doctor who has diagnosed breakfast as a hazard (at least for type 2 diabetics), so to help those type 2s survive breakfast (if they can't skip it) he has harnessed the second meal phenomenon.[6]

Glucose is not the only compound that can stimulate the islets of Langerhans to secrete insulin: some amino acids will too. And as we know, once it's been secreted insulin will inhibit the release of free fatty acids from the fat cells, so their blood levels will fall, and so the usual insulin-resistance of fasting will be reversed.

But amino acids do not damage the body the way glucose does, and Roy Taylor has shown that if a small protein snack is taken some time before the first meal of the day, the usual post-prandial hyperglycaemia is reduced. So if you've type 2 diabetes and if you simply can't skip breakfast, I'd recommend you eat a boiled egg (40p) or half a mozzarella (49p from Tesco) an hour before the first meal of the day. Ideally, though, you'd limit your breakfast to that egg or half mozzarella.

And if you've type 2 diabetes and if you *have* skipped breakfast (good for you!) your glucometer might tell you that eating an egg or half a mozzarella an hour before lunch might help keep blood sugar levels down after that meal too.

How do I, personally, live? On making my diagnosis of type 2, our family doctor prescribed various oral drugs for me, yet – initially – I nonetheless woke in the mornings with high blood glucose levels, often of 8–9 mmol/l. Only when I adopted a no-sugar, low-carbohydrate diet did these come down to around 7 mmol/l. But that was still too high, whereupon I discovered that if I went on a vegan diet, those early morning levels fell even further, down to 4–5.5 mmol/l, which are the normal levels and which thus confirmed that animal products aggravate my type 2.

Atrial fibrillation: The vegan diet had another benefit: it helped control my atrial fibrillation (AF). Two of the commonest medical conditions of men my age are type 2 diabetes and atrial fibrillation (I've a commonplace body) and the episodes of fibrillation (which is a condition when the heart beats irregularly) were a worry, because when I got them I could walk only 100 yards before losing my breath. But the vegan diet hugely reduced the incidence of episodes. AF is provoked by inflammation[7] – and animal products in their turn provoke inflammation – which presumably explains why a vegan diet helped reverse my condition.

Meat: I soon discarded my vegan diet, though, because – being also low-carbohydrate – it was boring (there's a limit to how many nuts and mushrooms this man can eat), but thanks to my glucometer I discovered that a white meat and fish and dairy diet (still low-carbohydrate of course) was reasonably good at keeping down my blood glucose levels (early morning blood glucose levels of 5.5–7) and at helping prevent AF episodes, which showed that red meat is the great enemy of my blood glucose levels and AF. Yet as I mentioned above, even non-red meat animal products must be doing some damage, so I keep my veganism in reserve, and when – as sometimes happens – my morning blood glucose levels start to run above 7, I revert to nuts and mushrooms for a day or two, whereupon those early morning levels soon return to the normal range.

Cholesterol: On abandoning my vegan diet I made yet another discovery: my blood cholesterol levels remained just fine. When I was initially diagnosed, my total cholesterol levels were worryingly high at 7.5 mmol/l (normal range up to 5), and though they came down on statins, I didn't respond well to those drugs, and it was only when I went low-carbohydrate and vegan that the LDL cholesterol levels came properly down (they now run around 4.5). But it transpired that my total (and indeed LDL) cholesterols don't care whether I'm doing a vegan diet or just a no-red meat diet; as long as I avoid red meat and carbohydrates, they're happy.

Alcohol: My doctor's third piece of dietary advice had been to avoid (or at least cut down on) alcohol. As usual he was only reiterating the official advice: in the words of the Mayo Clinic, which is one of the most respected medical bodies on the planet: 'Alcohol can worsen diabetes complications.'[8]

But on New Year's Day 2010 I'd given up – as was my custom – alcohol for January, yet (for no particular reason) I'd stayed on the wagon that year, so by mid-May I'd been teetotal for four and a half months. But that was the month my body chose to tip into frank diabetes, so I doubted that alcohol could be blamed for my problem. Initially I continued to abstain, yet one evening I succumbed to the demon drink, only to find my blood glucose level the following morning to be gloriously low. I've since drunk religiously every night, to very good blood glucose effect.

Which is hardly surprising, as the biochemists have known for decades that alcohol, on being metabolised, inhibits the liver's synthesis of glucose, which the diabetic charities have also long known: 'Drinking alcohol makes hypoglycaemia (low blood glucose levels) more likely,'[9] though in my case they've never fallen worryingly low, however much alcohol I've drunk in the interests of research.

Envoi

So there we have it, breakfast damages us in at least four different ways. First, it not only increases the numbers of calories we consume in the morning but, contrary to myth, it doesn't decrease *pari passu* the numbers of calories we eat at lunch. Second, it provokes hunger pangs later in the day, sometimes in the morning, sometimes in the afternoon, and sometimes both in the morning *and* in the afternoon. Third, because the morning is a time of natural insulin-resistance, eating then will help both provoke and aggravate the metabolic syndrome, which is the mass killer of our day. Which, fourth, is further aggravated by today's carbohydratisation of breakfast, which is generally a carbohydrate-laden meal.

I hope that we will soon embrace a new world, where eating breakfast is viewed as the privilege only of the slim, fit and young. For everyone else, I'm afraid, the mantra has to be an adaptation of Winston Churchill's 'one of the secrets of a happy marriage is never to see . . . the loved one before noon,'[1] namely:

not a calorie before noon.

Some of my friends complain that that is too austere a regime, and that a dash of milk in a morning cup of tea or coffee should be admissible, and of course it is. But if the goal is 'not a calorie before noon' then even a reprobate who does not move completely to a calorie-free morning should nonetheless achieve a health bonus.

Afterword

On 28 August 2016, the day after I delivered the final version of this book to the copy editors, I was alerted by a friend to a story in that day's *Daily Mail* headlined: 'Could six meals a day keep heart disease at bay? Regular eating found to reduce the chance of dying from clogged arteries by 30%'.

It wasn't hard to find the original paper, which had just been published by a team from Johns Hopkins University (a prestigious university in Baltimore, MD) in the *Annals of Epidemiology*, and which reported on the health of nearly 7,000 people who had been followed over fifteen years.[1] Some of those people happened to eat only once or twice a day, while others happened to eat up to six times a day; and those who ate more often, lived longer.

Yet those who lived longer differed in many ways from those who died earlier, including being older, more female, much whiter, much less black or Hispanic, and markedly better educated.

The authors tried to correct for these and other factors, but they obviously failed because the biology is so complex. Thus the six-times-a-day eaters ate 758 calories more every day than the two-times-a-day eaters, which is clearly unhealthy, so their longevity will have been despite – not because of – their eating breakfast and other gratuitous meals.

As I've noted before, this sort of study only confirms what Michael Marmot established long ago, namely that in the west the upper socio-economic groups outlive the lower groups by about seven years, probably because they experience less stress.[2] And since the upper groups tend to eat breakfast and other regular meals, while the lower groups tend to eat less regularly, the Johns Hopkins study had really only shown a correlation – not a causation – between frequent eating and longevity.

When I emailed the Johns Hopkins researchers, they were gracious enough to acknowledge that: 'This is an observational study,' so we couldn't know about actual cause-and-effect until someone had done 'a randomized controlled trial'. Which is why the *Daily Mail* might have done better to have headlined the article:

> 'Could six meals a day keep heart disease at bay? We don't know, but probably not'.

And with that final retrospect, I will finish this book.

References

Prologue

1 C.J. Rebello et al. (2016), 'Instant oatmeal increases satiety and reduces energy intake compared to a ready-to-eat oat-based breakfast cereal: a randomised crossover trial', *J Am Col Nutr* 35: 41–9.

1: My diagnosis

1 Diabetes UK (2013), *Annual Reports*, www.diabetes.org.uk/About-us/Annual-reports/.

2 Diabetes UK (2010), *Eating Well with Type 2 Diabetes*, http://www.diabetes.org.uk/upload/How%20we%20help/catalogue/EatingWell_T2.pdf. Accessed April 2015.

3 Diabetes.co.uk (2016), *NHS Diet Advice for Diabetes*. Accessed 15 October 2016.

4 American Diabetes Association (2014), *Annual Report, Strategic Plan, and Financials*, http://www.diabetes.org/about-us/who-we-are/reports.

5 American Diabetes Association (2014), *Recipes for Healthy Living*, www.diabetes.org/mfa-recipes/about-our-meals-plans.html. Accessed 12 December 2014.

6 Guido Freckmann et al. (2007), 'Continuous glucose profiles in healthy subjects under everyday life conditions and after different meals', *J Diabetes Sci Technol* 1: 695–703.

7 T. Parkner, J.K. Nielsen, T.D. Sandahl, B.M. Bibby, B.S. Jensen and J.S. Christiansen (2011), 'Do all patients with type 2 diabetes need breakfast?', *Eur J Clin Nutr* 65: 761–3. (A note: by convention, the name of the leader of a biological research group often goes last; conventions vary in different academic disciplines, so for example it is usual for authors of papers in economics to be ordered alphabetically.)

8 X.M. Chen et al. (2010), 'Correlation between glucose fluctuations and carotid intima-media thickness in type 2 diabetes', *Diabetes Res Clin Pract* 90: 95–9.

9 L. Monnier, C. Colette and D.R. Owens (2008), 'Glycemic variability: the third component of the dysglycemia in diabetes. Is it important? How to measure it?', *J Diabetes Sci Technol* 2: 1094–100.

10 NICE (December 2015), 'Type 2 diabetes in adults: management', www.nice.org.uk/guidance/ng28/chapter/1-Recommendations. Accessed 18 March 2016.

11 U.L. Malanda et al. (18 January 2012), 'Self-monitoring of blood glucose in patients with type 2 diabetes mellitus who are not using insulin', *Cochrane DB Syst Rev*, doi: 10.1002/14651858.CD005060. pub3.

12 C.D. Madigan et al. (2014), 'A randomised controlled trial of the effectiveness of self-weighing as a weight loss intervention', *Int J Behave Nutr Phys Act* 11: 125, doi:10.1186/s12966-014-0125-9.

13 J.J. VanWormer et al. (2012), 'Self-weighing frequency is associated with weight gain prevention over 2 years among working adults', *Int J Behav Med* 19: 351–8; D.M. Steinberg et al. (2013), 'The efficacy of a daily self-weighing weight loss intervention using smart scales and e mail', *Obesity* 21: 1789–97; M.L. Butryn et al. (2007), 'Consistency of self-monitoring of weight: a key component of successful weight-loss maintenance', *Obesity* 15: 3091–6; J.A. Linde et al. (2005), 'Self-weighing in weight gain prevention and weight loss trials', *Ann Behav Med* 30: 210–16; J.J. VanWormer at al. (2008), 'The impact of regular self-weighing in weight management: a systematic literature review', *Int J Behave Nutr Phys Act* 5: 54, doi:10.1186/1479-5868-5-54.

14 D.M. Bravata (2007), 'Using pedometers to increase physical activity and improve health: a systematic review', *J Am Med Assoc* 298: 2296–304.

15 Diabetes UK (April 2013), *Self Monitoring of Blood Glucose for Adults with Type 2 Diabetes*, www.diabetes.org.uk/Documents/ Position%20statements/Diabetes-UK-position-statement-SMBG-Type2-0413.pdf. Accessed 19 March 2016.

16 www.diabetes-book.com/. Accessed 14 March 2016.

2: The glorification of breakfast

1 Paraphrased from Homer, *The Iliad*, translated in 1898 by Samuel Butler, http://classics.mit.edu/Homer/iliad.19.xix.html.

2 Homer, *The Odyssey*, translated in 2004 by A.S. Kline, http://www. poetryintranslation.com/PITBR/Greek/Odyssey16.htm.

3 H.A. Anderson (2013), *Breakfast: A History*, Altamira, Lanham, New York, pp. 5, 8.

4 A. Barbero (2004), *Charlemagne: Father of a Continent*, University of Chicago Press, p. 121.

5 Garrick Mallery (July 1888), 'Manners and meals', *Am Anthropol* 196, quoted in H.A. Anderson (2013), *Breakfast: A History*, Altamira, Lanham, New York, p. 11.

6 Fordham University (Accessed 15 August 2015), *Modern History Sourcebook: William Harrison (1534–1593), Description of Elizabethan England* (from *Holinshed's Chronicles*), legacy.fordham.edu/halsall/mod/1577harrison-england.asp#Chapter%20VI.

7 Edmund Hollings (1602), *De salubri studiosorum victu*, quoted in Ken Albala (2002), 'Hunting for breakfast in medieval and early modern Europe', in Harlan Walker (ed.), *The Meal*, Prospect, Devon, UK.

8 Colin Spencer, *British Food*, p. 87, quoted in H.A. Anderson (2013), *Breakfast: A History*, Altamira, Lanham, New York, p. 11.

9 I. Mortimer (14 August 2015), 'How the Tudors invented breakfast', *History Extra*, www.historyextra.com/feature/tudors/how-tudors-invented-breakfast.

10 Thomas Cogan (1589), *The Haven of Health*, quoted in Ken Albala (2002), 'Hunting for breakfast in medieval and early modern Europe', in Harlan Walker (ed.), *The Meal*, Prospect, Devon, UK.

11 Margaret Lane (2005), 'Food', in Janet Todd (ed.), *Jane Austen in Context*, Cambridge University Press, p. 264.

12 M. Lane (1995), *Jane Austen and Food*, Hambledon Press, London, pp. 26–7.

13 A. Trollope (1875), *The Way We Live Now*, Chapman and Hall, London, p. 57.

14 Ibid., p. 31.

15 William Robertson (1847), *Treatise on Diet and Regimen*, 4th edn, John Churchill, London, pp. 288–9.

16 J.H. Kellogg (1881 edn), *Plain Facts for Old and Young*, Ayer Publishing, North Stratford, NH, pp. 294–6. At Project Gutenberg.

17 Ibid., p. 54.

18 Greg Jenner (2015), *A Million Years in a Day: A Curious History of Everyday Life*, Weidenfeld and Nicolson, London. Quoted by Greg Jenner (January 2015), 'Waking up with Plato', *BBC History Magazine*, p. 41.

19 Quoted in Edward Bernays, *Public Relations Wiki*, http://pr.wikia.com/wiki/Edward_Bernays. Accessed 31 March 2016.

20 www.youtube.com/watch?v=6vFz_FgGvJI. Accessed 20 October 2016.

21 Quoted in D. Mohammadi (26 March 2016), 'The great breakfast myth', *New Scientist*, No. 3066, p. 41.

22 William Robertson (1847), *Treatise on Diet and Regimen*, 4th edn, John Churchill, London, p. 285.

23 Adelle Davis Foundation, 'What She Said', www.adelledavis.org/adelle-davis/what-she-said/. Accessed October 2015.

24 Quoted in Joan Arehart-Treichel (1973), 'The great medical debate over low blood sugar', *Science News* 103: 172–4.

25 Ibid.

26 Ibid.

27 Ibid.

28 Elsa Orent-Keiles and Lois F. Hallman (1949), *The Breakfast Meal in Relation to Blood-Sugar Values*, United States Department of Agriculture, Washington, DC.

29 Ken Alabala (2003), *Food in Early Modern Europe*, Greenwood Press, Westport, CT, p. 233.

30 F. Marangoni et al. (2009), 'A consensus document on the role of breakfast in the attainment and maintenance of health and wellness', *Acta Biomed* 80: 166–71.

31 The easiest way of accessing this information is on the *Google* List of Countries by Life Expectancy page. Accessed 7 April 2016.

32 Quoted in I. Mortimer (April 2013), 'How the Tudors invented breakfast', *BBC History Magazine*, www.historyextra.com/feature/tudors/how-tudors-invented-breakfast.

33 D. Guthrie (1944), 'The breviary and dyetary of Andrew Boorde (1490–1549), physician, priest and traveller', *Proc R Soc Med* 37: 507–9.

34 Anne Charlton (2005), 'An example of health education in the early 17th century: *Naturall and Artificial Directions for Health* by William Vaughan', *Health Educ Res* 20: 656–64.

35 Quoted by F.J. Furnivall (1868), *Early English Meals and Manners*, Kegan Paul, London, p. 135.

36 Ibid., p. 141.

37 F. Kafka (1915), *Metamorphosis*, www.authorama.com/book/metamorphosis.html, paragraph 30. Translated in 2002 by David Wyllie.

38 A. Hunty et al. (2013), 'Does regular breakfast cereal consumption help children and adolescents stay slimmer? A systematic review and meta-analysis', *Obes Facts* 6: 70–85.

3: Breakfast in an age of commercial science

 1 Lenna F. Cooper (1917), in *Good Health*, 52. Quoted by S. Klein (7 October 2014), 'A brief history of how breakfast got its "healthy" rep', *Huffpost Healthy Living*, http://www.huffingtonpost.com/2014/10/06/breakfast-most-important-history_n_5910054.html.

2 Eric Schroeder (14 February 2014), 'Global breakfast cereal market to reach \$43.2 billion by 2019', *Food Business News*, http://www.foodbusinessnews.net/articles/news_home/Consumer_Trends/2014/02/Report_Global_breakfast_cereal.aspx?ID=%7B587FC363-F568-4088-B844-1A795384C7C0%7D&cck=1.

3 Daniel James (12 April 2014), 'Can rivals poach McDonald's breakfast business?', *Motley Fool*, http://www.fool.com/investing/general/2014/04/12/can-rivals-poach-away-mcdonalds-breakfast-business.aspx.

4 Kellogg's (2015), 'Kellogg's Special K Flatbread Breakfast Sandwich Sausage, Egg and Cheese', www.kelloggs.com/en_US/kelloggs-special-k-flatbread-sandwich-sausage-egg-and-cheese.html. Accessed 6 February 2015.

5 NHS Choices (19 June 2013), 'Salt: the facts', www.nhs.uk/Livewell/Goodfood/Pages/salt.aspx. Accessed 6 February 2015.

6 H. Stelfox et al. (1998), 'Conflict of interest in the debate over calcium-channel antagonists', *New Eng J Med* 338: 101–6.

7 L.I. Lesser, C.B. Ebbeling, M. Goozner, D. Wypij and D.S. Ludwig (2007), 'Relationship between funding source and conclusion among nutrition-related scientific articles', *PLOS Med* 4(1): e5, doi:10.1371/journal.pmed.0040005.

8 H.J. Leidy et al. (2013), 'Beneficial effects of a higher-protein breakfast on the appetitive, hormonal, and neural signals controlling energy intake regulation in overweight/obese, "breakfast skipping," late-adolescent girls', *Am J Clin Nutr* 97: 677–88.

9 The Beef Board, www.beefboard.org. Accessed July 2015.

10 N. Teicholz (2014), *The Big Fat Surprise*, Scribe, London.

11 J. Yudkin (2nd edn 1986, reprinted 2012), *Pure, White and Deadly*, Penguin, London.

12 A. Keys (1971), 'Sucrose in the diet and coronary heart disease', *Atherosclerosis* 14: 193–202.

13 T. Kealey (2008), *Sex, Science and Profits*, William Heinemann, London.

14 T.P. Stossel (2015), *Pharmaphobia: How the Conflict of Interest Myth Undermines American Medical Innovation*, Rowman & Littlefield, Lanham, MD.

4: Myth No. 1: Breakfast cereals are healthy

1 Which? (2006), *Cereal Re-offenders*, http://www.which.co.uk/documents/pdf/cereal-reoffenders-which-report-176973.pdf.

2 F. Lawrence (2008), *Eat Your Heart Out*, Penguin, London.

3 K. Rajakumar (2000), 'Pellagra in the United States: a historical perspective', *South Med J* 93: 272–7.

4 L.A. Berner et al. (2014), 'Fortified foods are major contributors to nutrient intakes in diets of US children and adolescents', *J Acad Nutr Diet* 114: 1009–22.

5 W. Sichert-Hellert and M. Kersting (2003), 'Impact of fortified breakfast cereals on iron intake in German children and adolescents', *J Paed Gastr Nutr* 36: 149–53.

6 D. Lodge (1975), *Changing Places*, Martin Secker and Warburg, London, p. 172.

7 www.euromonitor.com/breakfast-cereals-in-the-us/report. Accessed 8 March 2016. See also S. Strom (10 September 2014), 'Cereals begin to lose their snap, crackle and pop', *New York Times*.

8 R.G. Thomas et al. (2013), 'Recent trends in ready-to-eat breakfast cereals in the US', *Proc Food Sci* 2: 20–26.

9 H. Brussow (2013), 'Nutrition, population growth and disease: a short history of lactose', *Environ Microbiol* 15: 2154–61.

10 D.A. Savaiano (2014), 'Lactose digestion from yogurt: mechanism and relevance', *Am J Clin Nutr* 99 (5 Suppl): 1251S–5S.

11 Andrew Prentice (2014), 'Dairy products in global public health', *Am J Clin Nutr* 99 (suppl): 1212S–16S.

5: Myth No. 2: Breakfast is good for the brain

1 A. Hoyland, L. Dye and C.L. Laewton (2009), 'A systematic review of the effect of breakfast on the cognitive performance of children and adolescents', *Nutr Res Rev* 22: 220–43; Ernesto Pollitt and Rebecca Mathews (1998), 'Breakfast and cognition: an integrative summary', *Am J Clin Nutr* 67 (suppl): 804S–13S.

2 A.P. Smith, A.M. Kendrick and A.L. Maben (1992), 'Effects of breakfast and caffeine on performance and mood in the late morning and after lunch', *Neuropsychobiology* 26: 198–204.

3 A. Smith et al. (1994), 'Effects of breakfast and caffeine on cognitive performance, mood and cardiovascular functioning', *Appetite* 22: 39–55.

4 Valeria Edefonti et al. (2014), 'The effect of breakfast composition and energy contribution on cognitive and academic performance: a systematic review', *Am J Clin Nutr* 100: 626–56.

5 D. de Ridder et al. (23 October 2014), 'Always gamble on an empty stomach: hunger is associated with advantageous decision making', *PLOS One* 9(10): 10.1371/journal.pone.0111081.

6 H.A. Anderson (2013), *Breakfast: A History*, Altamira, Lanham, New York, p. 155.

7 Albert Shaw (1891), 'Food aided education: experiments in Paris, London and Birmingham', *Review of Reviews*, New York, quoted by

H.A. Anderson (2013), *Breakfast: A History*, Altamira, Lanham, New York, p. 154.

8 Huey Newton (2002), 'Hoover and the FBI', PBS, http://www.pbs. org/hueypnewton/people/people_hoover.html. Nik Heynen (2009), 'Bending the bars of empire from every ghetto for survival', *Ann Assoc Am Geogr*, http://nheynen.myweb.uga.edu/pdf/Annals, quoted by H.A. Anderson (2013), *Breakfast: A History*, Altamira, Lanham, New York, p. 155.

6: Myth No. 3: Breakfast is slimming

1 J.M. de Castro (2004), 'The time of day of food intake influences overall intake in humans', *J Nutr* 134: 104–11.

2 D.A. Levitsky and C.R. Pacanowski (2 July 2013), 'Effect of skipping breakfast on subsequent energy intake', *Physiol Behav* 119: 9–16, doi: 10.1016/j.physbeh.2013.05.006. Epub 11 May 2013.

3 G.C. Rampersaud, M.A. Pereira, B.L. Girard, J. Adams and J.D. Metzl (2005), 'Breakfast habits, nutritional status, body weight, and academic performance in children and adolescents', *J Am Diet Assoc* 105: 743–60.

4 V. Schusdziarra et al. (2011), 'Impact of breakfast on daily energy intake – an analysis of absolute versus relative breakfast calories', *Nutr J* 10: 5, http://www.nutritionj.com/content/10/1/5.

5 Quoted from Brian Wansink (2006), *Mindless Eating*, Bantam Dell, New York, p. 176. The references to the original work of Birch and Fisher are:- L.L. Birch et al. (1987), 'Clean up your plate: effects of child feeding practices on the conditioning of meal size', *Learn Motiv* 18: 301–17; L.L. Birch and J.O. Fisher (2000), 'Mother's child-feeding practices influence daughters' eating and weight', *Am J Clin Nutr* 71: 1054–61; J.O. Fisher et al. (2003), 'Children's bite size and intake of entree are greater with large portions than with age-appropriate or self-selected portions', *Am J Clin Nutr* 77: 1164–70.

6 M. May (2011), *Eat What You Love, Love What You Eat*, Nourish Publishing, Independent Publishers Group, Chicago, IL.

7 E. Robinson et al. (2013), 'Eating attentively: a systematic review and meta-analysis of the effect of food intake memory and awareness on eating', *Am J Clin Nutr*, doi: 10.3945/ajcn.112. 045245.

8 J.M. de Castro (1995), 'Social facilitation and inhibition of eating', in B.M. Marriot (ed.), *Not Eating Enough: Overcoming Underconsumption of Military Operational Rations*, National Academies Press (US).

9 Brian Wansink (2006), *Mindless Eating*, Bantam Dell, New York, p. 99.

10 J.M. de Castro (1995), 'Social facilitation and inhibition of eating', in B.M. Marriot (ed), *Not Eating Enough: Overcoming Underconsumption of Military Operational Rations*, National Academies Press (US).

11 T. Doring and B. Wansink (28 December 2015), 'The waiter's weight: does a server's BMI relate to how much food diners order?', *Environ Behav*, doi: 10.1177/001391651561108.

12 D. Mori et al. (1987), 'Eating lightly and the self-presentation of femininity', *J Pers Soc Psychol* 53: 693–702.

7: Yo-yo dieting

1 G.C. Rampersaud, M.A. Pereira, B.L. Girard, J. Adams and J.D. Metzl (2005), 'Breakfast habits, nutritional status, body weight, and academic performance in children and adolescents', *J Am Diet Assoc* 105: 743–60.

2 Mary E. Shaw (1998), 'Adolescent breakfast skipping: an Australian study', *Adolescence* 33: 851–61.

3 B.M. Malinauskas et al. (2006), 'Dieting practices, weight perceptions, and body composition: a comparison of normal weight, overweight and obese college females', *Nutr J* 5: 11, doi:10.1186/1475-2891-5-11.

4 G.C. Rampersaud, M.A. Pereira, B.L. Girard, J. Adams and J.D. Metzl (2005), 'Breakfast habits, nutritional status, body weight, and academic performance in children and adolescents', *J Am Diet Assoc* 105: 743–60.

5 J.W. Anderson et al. (2001), 'Long-term weight loss maintenance: a meta analysis of US studies', *Am J Clin Nutr* 74: 579–84.

6 M. McGuire et al. (1999), 'Behavioral strategies of individuals who have maintained long-term weight losses', *Obesity Res* 7: 334–41.

7 A. Bosy-Westphal et al. (2013), 'Effect of weight loss and regain on adipose tissue distribution, composition of lean mass and resting energy expenditure in young overweight and obese adults', *Int J Obes* 37: 1371–7.

8 A.G. Dulloo et al. (2006), 'The thrifty "catch-up fat" phenotype: its impact on insulin sensitivity during growth trajectories to obesity and metabolic syndrome', *Int J Obes* 30: S23–S35.

9 K.D. Tipton and R.R. Wolfe (2001), 'Exercise, protein metabolism, and muscle growth', *Int J Sport Nutr Exerc Metab* 11: 109–32. See also T.M. Longland et al. (27 January 2016). 'Higher compared with lower dietary protein during an energy deficit combined with intense exercise promotes greater lean mass gain and fat mass loss: a randomised trial', *Am J Clin Nutr*, doi: 10.3945/ajcn.115.119339.

10 M. Rosenbaum and R.L. Leibel (2010), 'Adaptive thermogenesis in humans', *Int J Obes (Lond)* 34: S47–S55.

11 N.D. Knuth et al. (2014), 'Metabolic adaptation following massive weight loss is related to the degree of energy imbalance and changes in circulating leptin', *Obesity* 22: 2563–9.

12 H.R. Wyatt et al. (1999), 'Resting energy expenditure in reduced-obese subjects in the National Weight Control Registry', *Am J Clin Nutr* 69: 1189–93.

13 M. Rosenbaum et al. (2008), 'Long-term persistence of adaptive thermogenesis in subjects who have maintained a reduced body weight', *Am J Clin Nutr* 88: 906–12.

14 P. Sumathran et al. (2011), 'Long-term persistence of hormonal adaptations to weight loss', *New Eng J Med* 365: 1597–1604. E.W. Iepsen et al. suggest, though, that after a year, some key appetite hormones revert to pre-diet levels (E.W. Iepsen et al. (14 March 2016), 'Successful weight loss maintenance includes long-term increased meal responses of GLP-1 PYY 3-36', *Eur J Endocrinol*, doi: 10.1530/EJE-15-1116).

15 T. Spector (2015), *The Diet Myth*, Weidenfeld and Nicolson, London, p. 11.

16 D.B. Allison et al. (1996), 'The heritability of body mass index among an international sample of monozygotic twins reared apart', *Int J Obes* 20: 501–6.

17 T. Spector (2015), *The Diet Myth*, Weidenfeld and Nicolson, London, p. 6.

18 K.H. Pietilainen et al. (2012), 'Does dieting make you fat? A twin study', *Int J Obes (Lond)* 36: 456–64.

19 A.G. Dulloo et al. (2015), 'How dieting makes the lean fatter: from a perspective of body composition autoregulation through adipostats and proteinstats awaiting discovery', *Obesity Rev* 16: 25–35.

8: Chaotic lives

1 A. Keski-Rahkonen, J. Kaprio, A. Rissanen, M. Virkkunen and R.J. Rose (2003), 'Breakfast skipping and health-compromising behaviors in adolescents and adults', *Eur J Clin Nutr* 57: 842–53.

2 H.M. Niemeier, H.A. Raynor, E.E. Lloyd-Richardson, M.L. Rogers and R.R. Wing (2006), 'Fast food consumption and breakfast skipping: predictors of weight gain from adolescence to adulthood in a nationally representative sample', *J Adolescent Health* 39: 842–9.

3 Mark Pereira at al. (2005), 'Fast food habits, weight gain, and insulin resistance (the CARDIA study): 15-year prospective analysis', *Lancet* 365: 36–42.

4 Quote from the National Institutes of Health's press release on Dr Pereira's paper (30 December 2004), www.nih.gov/news/pr/dec 2004/nhlbi-30.htm. Accessed September 2015.

5 Clare J. Seamark and Denis J. Periera Gray (1998), 'Teenagers and risk-taking: pregnancy and smoking', *Brit J Gen Prace* 48: 985–6.

6 Reuters (Tokyo, Friday, 26 December 2008, 4:26 p.m. IST), 'Japan teens skipping breakfast have sex younger', http://in.reuters.com/ article/2008/12/26/us-japan-sex-idINTRE4BP18P20081226.

7 T. Greenhalgh (1997), 'How to read a paper: getting your bearings; deciding what the paper is about', *BMJ* 315: 243–6.

9: Five breakfast sagas

1 Yunsheng Ma, Elizabeth R. Bertone, Edward J. Stanek III, George W. Reed, James R. Hebert, Nancy L. Cohen, Philip A. Merriam and Ira S. Ockene (2003), 'Association between eating patterns and obesity in a free-living US adult population', *Am J Epidemiol* 158: 85–92.

2 P.G. Lindqvist et al. (2014), 'Avoidance of sun exposure is a risk factor for all-cause mortality: results from the Melanoma in Southern Sweden cohort', *J Intern Med* 276: 77–86.

3 American Academy of Pediatrics, Task Force on Infant Sleep Position and Sudden Infant Death Syndrome (2000), 'Changing concepts of sudden infant death syndrome: implications for infant sleeping environment and sleep position', *Pediatrics* 105: 650–56.

4 Marcelle Pick (2015), 'The history of hormone replacement therapy (HRT) women to women', www.womentowomen.com/bioidenticals-and-hrt/history-of-hormone-replacement-therapy-hrt/. Accessed September 2015.

5 Elizabeth Siegel Watkins (2007), *The Estrogen Elixir: A History of Hormone Replacement Therapy in America*, Johns Hopkins University Press, Baltimore.

6 Berit Lilienthal Heitmann and Lauren Lissner (1995), 'Dietary underreporting by obese individuals – is it specific or non-specific?', *BMJ* 311: 986–9.

7 P.V. Dialektakou and P. Vranas (2008), 'Breakfast skipping and body mass index among adolescents in Greece: whether an association exists depends on how breakfast skipping is defined', *J Am Diet Assoc* 108: 1517–25.

8 buyonboard.easyjet.com. Accessed March 2015.

9 James A. Betts et al. (2014), 'The causal role of breakfast in energy balance and health: a randomized controlled trial in lean adults', *Am J Clin Nutr* 100: 539–47.

10 Anna Hodgekiss (2014), 'Breakfast might not be the most important meal of the day after all', *Daily Mail*, http://www.dailymail.co.uk/health/article-2733767/Breakfast-NOT-important-meal-day-Scientists-not-kickstart-metabolism-aid-weight-loss.html#ixzz3FUfKcnED.

11 E.A. Chowdhury et al. (10 February 2016), 'The causal role of breakfast in energy balance and health: a randomized controlled trial in obese people', *Am J Clin Nutr*, doi: 10.3945/ajcn.115.122044.

12 Iona Merikanto et al. (2013), 'Associations of chronotype and sleep with cardiovascular diseases and type 2 diabetes', *Chronobiol Int* 30: 470–77.

13 Sirimon Reutrakul et al. (2014), 'The relationship between breakfast skipping, chronotype, and glycemic control in type 2 diabetes', *Chronobiol Int* 31: 64–71.

14 M. Wittmann, J. Dinich, M. Merrow and T. Roenneberg (2006), 'Social jetlag: misalignment of biological and social time', *Chronobiol Int* 23: 497–509.

15 Ilona Merikanto et al. (2013), 'Associations of chronotype and sleep with cardiovascular diseases and type 2 diabetes', *Chronobiol Int* 30: 470–77.

16 Sirimon Reutrakul et al. (2014), 'The relationship between breakfast skipping, chronotype, and glycemic control in type 2 diabetes', *Chronobiol Int* 31: 64–71.

17 Norito Kawakami, Naoyoshi Takatsuka and Hiroyuki Shimizu (2004), 'Sleep disturbance and onset of type 2 diabetes', *Diabetes Care* 27: 282–3.

18 P.S. Hogenkamp et al. (2013), 'Acute sleep deprivation increases portion size and affects food choice in young men', *Psychoneuroendocrinology* 38: 1668–74.

19 J.L. Broussard et al. (2015), 'Sleep restriction increases free fatty acids in healthy men', *Diabetologia*, doi 10.1007/s00125-015-3500-4.

20 A.N. Vgontzas et al. (2005), 'Daytime napping after a night of sleep loss decreases sleepiness, improves performance, and causes beneficial changes in cortisol and interleukin-6 secretion', *Am J Physiol Endocrinol Metab* 292: E253–61.

21 S. Kanazawa and K. Perina (2009), 'Why night owls are more intelligent', *Person Indiv Differ* 47: 685–90, doi:10.1016/j.paid.2009.05.021.

22 H. Szajewska and M. Ruszczynski (2010), 'Systematic review demonstrating that breakfast consumption influences body weight outcomes in children and adolescents in Europe', *Crit Rev Food Sci Nutr* 50: 113–19.

10: The Harvard and Cambridge challenges

1 A.A.W.A. van der Heijden, F.B. Hu, E.B. Rimm and R.M. van Dam (2007), 'A prospective study of breakfast consumption and weight gain among US men', *Obesity* 15: 2463–9.

2 R.A. Mekary, E. Giovannucci, W. Willett, R. van Dam and F. Hu (2012), 'Eating pattern and type 2 diabetes risk in men: breakfast omission, eating frequency, and snacking'. *Am J Clin Nutr* 95: 1182–9.

3 Leah E. Cahill, Stephanie E. Chiuve, Rania A. Mekary, Majken K. Jensen, Alan J. Flint, Frank B. Hu and Eric B. Rimm (2013), 'Prospective study of breakfast eating and incident coronary heart disease in a cohort of male US health professionals', *Circulation* 128: 337–43.

4 N.K. Valtora et al. (2016), 'Loneliness and social isolation as risk factors for coronary heart disease and stroke: systematic review and meta-analysis of longitudinal observational studies', *Heart* 102: 1009–16.

5 A. Mirzaei et al. (2016), 'Social cognitive predictors of breakfast consumption in primary school's male students', *Globl J Health Sci* 8: 124–32.

6 A.A.W.A. van der Heijden, F.B. Hu, E.B. Rimm and R.M. van Dam (2007), 'A prospective study of breakfast consumption and weight gain among US men', *Obesity* 15: 2463–9.

7 http://forums.texags.com/main/forum.reply.asp?topic_id=2334915& forum_id=48
http://www.forbes.com/sites/alicegwalton/2013/07/23/why-is-skipping-breakfast-so-bad-for-our-heart-health/.

8 www.bbc.co.uk/news/health-23403744. Accessed 7 January 2016.

9 L.R. Purslow et al. (2008), 'Energy intake at breakfast and weight change: prospective study of 6,764 middle aged men and women', *Am J Epidemiol* 167: 188–92.

10 H.R. Farshchi et al. (2005), 'Deleterious effects of omitting breakfast on insulin sensitivity and fasting lipid profiles in healthy lean women', *Am J Clin Nutr* 81: 388–96.

11 D. Zeevi et al. (2015), 'Personalized nutrition by prediction of glycemic responses', *Cell* 163: 1079–94.

12 C. Bouchard et al. (1990), 'The response to long-term overfeeding in identical twins', *N Engl J Med* 322: 1477–82.

13 N.M. Astbury et al. (2011), 'Breakfast consumption affects appetite, energy intake, and the metabolic and endocrine responses to foods consumed later in the day', *J Nutr* 141: 1381–9.

11: The heroic breakfast guerrillas

1 A.W. Brown, M.M. Bohan Brown and D.B. Allison (2013), 'Belief beyond the evidence: Using the proposed effect of breakfast on obesity to show 2 practices that distort scientific evidence', *Am J Clin Nutr* 98: 1298–308.

2 R.A. Mekary and E. Giovannucci (2014), 'Belief beyond the evidence: Using the proposed effect of breakfast on obesity to show 2 practices that distort scientific evidence', *Am J Clin Nutr* 2014 Jan; 99(1): 212–3.

3 A.W. Brown, M.M. Bohan Brown and D.B. Allison (2014), 'Reply to R.A. Mekary and E. Giovannucci' *Am J Clin Nutr* 99: 213.

4 Emily J. Dhurandhar et al. (2014), 'The effectiveness of breakfast recommendations on weight loss: a randomized controlled trial', *Am J Clin Nutr* 100: 507–13.

5 D.G. Schlundt et al. (1992), 'The role of breakfast in the treatment of obesity: a randomised clinical trial', *Am J Clin Nutr* 55: 645–51.

6 D. Levitsky (2014), 'Next will be apple pie', *Am J Clin Nutr* 100: 503–4.

7 M. Chen et al. (2014), 'Dairy consumption and risk of type 2 diabetes: 3 cohorts of US adults and an updated meta-analysis', *BMC Medicine* 12: 215, doi:10.1186/s12916-014-0215-1.

8 H. Wu et al. (5 January 2015), 'Association between dietary whole grain intake and risk of mortality', *JAMA Int Med*, doi:10.1001/jamainternmed.2014.6283.

9 P.A. van den Brandt and L.J. Schouten (11 June 2015), 'Relationship of tree nut, peanut and peanut butter intake with total and cause-specific mortality: a cohort study and meta-analysis', *Int J Epidemiol*, doi: 10.1093/ije/dyv039.

10 M.L. Beroia et al. (28 January 2016), 'Dietary flavonoid intake and weight maintenance: three prospective cohorts of 124,086 US men and women followed for up to 24 years', *BMJ*, 352 dx.doi.org/10.1136/bmj.i17.

11 Editorial (2013), 'Shades of Grey', *Nature* 487: 410. Virginia Hughes (2013), 'The big fat truth', *Nature* 487: 428–30.

12 US Department of Agriculture and US Department of Health and Human Services (2010), *Dietary Guidelines for Americans, 2010*, US Government Printing Office, Washington, DC, https://health.gov/dietaryguidelines/dga2010/DietaryGuidelines2010.pdf, page 19.

13 P. Whoriskey (10 August 2015), 'The science of skipping breakfast: how government nutritionists may have gotten it wrong', *Washington Post*, www.washingtonpost.com/news/wonk/wp/2015/08/10/ the-science-of-skipping-breakfast-how-government-nutritionists-may-have-gotten-it-wrong/?tid=a_inl.

12: Blood glucose and breakfast: the unhealthy majority

1   R. Peter et al. (2009), 'Daytime variability of postprandial glucose tolerance and pancreatic B-cell function using 12-h profiles in persons with Type 2 diabetes', *Diabetic Med* 27: 266–73. Although this study did indeed report on twelve-hour profiles, dinner was eaten only four hours after lunch, so it was eaten earlier than in other studies: I don't think that is of importance, but in the case of discrepancies between studies, it should be noted.

2   L. Monnier et al. (2013), 'Magnitude of the dawn phenomenon and its impact on the overall glucose exposure in type 2 diabetes', *Diabetes Care* 36: 4057–62.

3   H. Fernemark et al. (2013), 'A randomised cross-over trial of the postprandial effects of three different diets in patients with type 2 diabetes', *PLOS One* 8: e79324, doi:10.1371/journal/pone.0079324. In this study, patients were given a true 'Mediterranean-style lunch', which included a glass of wine. Since alcohol can lower blood glucose levels (see later chapters), Dr Guldbrand introduced not one but two variables into his experiment, which makes it hard to isolate the relative effects of breakfast skipping and alcohol consumption in improving his patients' metabolism: they both contributed, and that's as much as we can say.

4   G. Boden, X. Chen and J. Urbain (1996), 'Evidence for a circadian rhythm of insulin sensitivity in patients with NIDDM caused by cyclic changes in hepatic glucose production', *Diabetes* 45: 1044–50. Later in this book I shall be showing how blood glucose levels rise because of skeletal muscle insulin-resistance, but hepatic insulin-resistance may be an even more important cause of that (G. Perriello et al. (1997), 'Evidence of increased systemic glucose production and gluconeogenesis in an early stage of NIDDM', *Diabetes* 43: 1010–16).

5   M.L. dos Santos et al. (2006), 'Daytime variations in glucose tolerance in people with impaired glucose tolerance', *Diabetes Res Clin Pract* 74: 257–62.

6   K.S. Polonsky et al. (1988), 'Twenty-four-hour profiles and pulsatile patterns of insulin secretion in normal and obese subjects', *J Clin Invest* 81: 442–8.

7   D. Jakubowicz et al. (2015), 'High-energy breakfast with low-energy dinner decreases overall daily hyperglycaemia in type 2 diabetic patients: a randomised clinical trial', *Diabetologia*, doi 10.1007/s00125-015-3524-9.

8   D. Jakubowicz et al. (2015), 'Fasting until noon triggers increased postprandial hyperglycaemia and impaired insulin response after lunch and dinner in individuals with type 2 diabetes: a randomized

clinical trial', *Diabetes Care* 38: 1820–26. These experiments were conducted over seventy-two hours, during which the breakfast skippers' intake was reduced from 2,100 to 1,400 calories a day, and since the recommended guidelines are 2,200 calories a day for men and 1,600 for women (which averages at 1,900 calories a day) and since half of the patients were men and half women, the patients were on a 25 per cent caloric restricted diet.

9 www.aftau.org/weblog-medicine--health?&storyid4704=2218&ncs 4704=3. Accessed 5 January 2016.

10 Scientific Advisory Committee on Nutrition (2011), *Dietary Reference Values for Energy*, TSO, London. www.gov.uk/ government/uploads/system/uploads/attachment_data/file/339317/ SACN_Dietary_Reference_Values_For_Energy.pdf.

11 D. Jakubowicz et al. (2013), 'High caloric intake at breakfast vs dinner differentially influences weight loss of overweight and obese women', *Obesity* 21: 2504–12.

12 M. Lombardo et al. (2014), 'Morning meal more efficient for fat loss in a 3-month lifestyle intervention', *J Am Coll Nutr* 33: 198–205.

13: Blood glucose and breakfast: the healthy minority

1 C. Malherbe et al. (1969), 'Circadian rhythms of blood sugar and plasma insulin levels in man', *Diabetologia* 5: 397–404.

2 K.S. Polonsky, B.D. Given and E. Van Cauter (1988), 'Twenty-Four-Hour Profiles and Pulsatile Patterns of Insulin Secretion in Normal and Obese Subjects', *J. Clin Invest* 81: 442–8.

3 Guido Freckmann et al. (2007), 'Continuous glucose profiles in healthy subjects under everyday life conditions and after different meals', *J Diabetes Sci Technol* 1: 695–703.

4 Jian Zhou et al. (2009), 'Reference values for continuous glucose monitoring in Chinese subjects', *Diabetes Care* 32: 1188–93.

5 Professor Taylor fed his subject 646 calories in the morning, but 858 calories at lunchtime. A. Jovanovic et al. (2009), 'The second-meal phenomenon is associated with enhanced muscle glycogen storage in humans', *Clin Sci* 117: 119–27.

6 T. Ruge et al. (2009), 'Fasted to fed trafficking of fatty acids in human adipose tissue reveals a novel regulatory step for enhanced fat storage', *J Clin Endocrinol Metab* 94: 1781–8.

7 E. Van Cauter et al. (1992), 'Circadian modulation of glucose and insulin responses to meals: relationship to cortisol rhythm', *Am J Physiol* 262: E467–75.

8 L.M. Morgan et al. (1999), 'Diurnal variations in peripheral insulin

resistance and plasma nonesterified fatty acid concentration: a possible link?', *Ann Clin Biochem* 36: 447–50.

9 Ahmed Saad et al. (2012), 'Diurnal pattern to insulin secretion and insulin action in healthy individuals', *Diabetes* 61: 2691–700. Note: the lead (last author) was Ananda Basu.

10 J.L. Broussard et al. (2015), 'Sleep restriction increases free fatty acids in healthy men', *Diabetologia*, doi 10.1007/s00125-015-3500-4. This was a study on four hours' sleep deprivation, which will be longer than that precipitated by Dr Polonsky, but the trends will be there.

11 R.S. Bienso et al. (2012), 'GLUT4 and glycogen synthase are key players in bed rest-induced insulin resistance', *Diabetes* 61: 1090–99.

12 James Norman (2016), 'Diagnosing diabetes', *Endocrineweb*, www.endocrineweb.com/conditions/diabetes/diagnosing-diabetes. Accessed 5 April 2016.

14: Why have the scientists claimed breakfast to be safe?

1 J.P.A.Ioannidis (2005), *Public Library of Science Medicine* 2(8): e124.

2 M.R. Rank and T.A. Hirschl (2009), 'Estimating the risk of food stamp use and impoverishment during childhood', *Arch Pediatr Adolesc Med* 163: 994–9.

3 T. Kealey (2008), *Sex, Science and Profits*, William Heinemann, London.

4 M. Nestle (3rd edn 2013), *Food Politics: How the Food Industry Influences Nutrition and Health*, University of California Press, p. 3.

15: The fat saga

1 A. Keys (1953), 'Atherosclerosis: a problem in newer public health', *J Mount Sinai Hospital* 2: 118–39.

2 A. Keys et al. (1955), 'Effects of diet on blood lipids in man, particularly cholesterol and lipoproteins', *Clin Chem* 1: 34–52.

3 J. Yudkin (2nd edn 1986, reprinted 2012), *Pure, White and Deadly*, Penguin, London, p. 86. J. Yudkin (1957), 'Diet and coronary thrombosis: hypothesis and fact', *Lancet* II: 155.

4 A. Grontved and F.B. Hu (2011), 'Television watching and risk of type 2 diabetes, cardiovascular disease and all-cause mortality: a meta-analysis', *JAMA* 305: 2448–55.

5 J. Yudkin (2nd edn 1986, reprinted 2012), *Pure, White and Deadly*, Penguin, London, p. 63.

6 J. Yerushalmy and H. Hilleboe (1957), 'Fat in the diet and mortality from heart disease: a methodological note', *N Y State J Medicine* 57:

2343–54. Quoted by N. Teicholz (2014), *Big Fat Surprise*, Scribe, London, p. 34.

7 See the review in E.H. Aherns Jr (1986), 'Carbohydrates, plasma triglycerides, and coronary heart disease', *Nutr Rev* 44: 60–64.

8 G. Mann et al. (1964), 'Cardiovascular disease in the Masai', *J Atheroscler Res* 4: 289–312.

9 A. Keys (1971), 'Sucrose in the diet and coronary heart disease', *Atherosclerosis* 14: 193–202.

10 A. Keys (ed.) (1970), 'Coronary heart disease in seven countries', *Circulation* 41 (4 Suppl): 1–200; A. Keys (ed.) (1980), *Seven Countries: A Multivariate Analysis of Death and Coronary Heart Disease*, Harvard University Press, Cambridge, MA. Both quoted by N. Teicholz (2014), *Big Fat Surprise*, Scribe, London, p. 38.

11 A. Menotti et al. (1999), 'Food intake patterns and 25-year mortality from coronary heart disease: cross-cultural correlations in the seven countries study', *Eur J Epidemiol* 15: 507–15.

12 For a list of these early clinical trials that did not confirm the Keys hypothesis, see N. Teicholz (2014), *Big Fat Surprise*, Scribe, London, p. 57.

13 R.H. Lustig (2012), in J. Yudkin, *Pure, White and Deadly*, Penguin, London, p. ix.

14 American Medical Association (1977,) 'Dietary goals for the United States: statement of the American Medical Association to the Select Committee on Nutrition and Human Needs, United States Senate', *R I Med J* 60: 576–81.

15 Zoe Harcombe at al. (2015), 'Evidence from randomised controlled trials did not support the introduction of dietary fat guidelines in 1977 and 1983: a systematic review and meta-analysis', *Open Heart* 2, doi10.1136/openhrt-2014-000196.

16 E.S. Gordon et al. (1963), 'A new concept in the treatment of obesity', *JAMA* 186: 156–66.

17 F.F. Samaha et al. (2003), 'A low-carbohydrate as compared with a low-fat diet on severe obesity', *New Engl J Med* 348: 2074–81; G.D. Foster et al. (2003), 'A randomized trial of a low-carbohydrate diet for obesity' *New Engl J Med* 348: 2082–90.

18 R. Estruch et al. (2013), 'Primary prevention of cardiovascular disease with a Mediterranean diet', *N Engl J Med* 368, doi: 10.1056/NEJMoa1200303.

19 F.L. Santos et al. (2012), 'Systematic review and meta-analysis of clinical trials of the effects of low carbohydrate diets in cardiovascular risk factors', *Obes Res* 13: 1048–66.

20 J.E. Muller et al. (2011), 'Carbohydrate restricted diet in conjunction with metformin and liraglutide is an effective treatment in patients with

deteriorated type 2 diabetes mellitus: proof-of-concept study', *Nutr Metabol* 8: 92, http://nutritionandmetabolism.com/content/ 8/1/92.

21 J.S. Volek et al. (2009), 'Carbohydrate restriction has a more favorable impact on the metabolic syndrome than a low fat diet', *Lipids* 44: 297–309.

22 A. Accurso et al. (2008), 'Dietary restriction in type 2 diabetes mellitus and metabolic syndrome: time for a critical appraisal', *Nutr Metab (Lond)* 5: 9, doi:10.1186/1743-7075-5-9.

23 C.D. Gardner (2007), 'Comparison of the Atkins, Zone, Ornish, and LEARN diets for change in weight and elated risk factors among overweight premenopausal women: the A TO Z weight loss study; a randomised trial', *JAMA* 297: 969–77.

24 E.A. Hu et al. (2012), 'White rice consumption and risk of type 2 diabetes: meta-analysis and systematic review', *BMJ* 344: e1454.

25 B. Senauer and M. Gemma (2006), 'Why is the obesity rate so low in Japan and high in the US? Some possible economic explanations', Ageconsearch.umn.edu/bitstream/14321/1/tr06-02s.pdf. Accessed 7 January 2016.

26 www.idf.org/membership/wp/japan. Accessed 7 January 2016.

27 A. Nanri et al. (2010), 'Rice intake and type 2 diabetes in Japanese men and women: The Japanese Public Health Center-based Prospective Study', *Am J Clin Nutr* 92: 1468–77.

28 NHS Choices (14/12/2014), 'Eight tips for healthy eating', http://www.nhs.uk/livewell/goodfood/eight-tips-healthy-eating.aspx. Accessed April 2015.

29 NHS Choices (31/03/2015), 'Starchy foods and carbohydrates', http://www.nhs.uk/Livewell/Goodfood/Pages/starchy-foods.aspx. Accessed April 2015.

30 *Dietary Guidelines for Americans, 2010*, p. 15, www.health.gov/dietaryguidelines/dga2010/DietaryGuidelines2010.pdf.

31 Diabetes UK (February 2013), *Diabetic Foods*, www.diabetes.org.uk/Documents/Position%/20statements/Diabetes-UK-position-statement-Diabetic-foods-0213.pdf. Accessed 26 March 2016.

32 American Diabetes Association (1995–2016), *Diabetes Myths*, www.diabetes.org/diabetes-basics-myths/. Accessed 26 March 2016.

33 American Diabetes Association (2014), *Carbohydrate Counting*, http://www.diabetes.org/food-and-fitness/food/what-can-i-eat/understanding-carbohydrates/carbohydrate-counting.html.

34 K.-T. Khaw (2001), 'Glycated haemoglobin, diabetes, and mortality in men in Norfolk cohort of European Prospective Investigation of Cancer and Nutrition (EPIC-Norfolk)', *BMJ* 322: 1–6.

35 W. Osler and T. McCrae (1923), *The Principles and Practice of Medicine*, Appleton and Co, New York. Quoted by W.S. Yancy Jr

et al. (2005), 'A low-carbohydrate, ketogenic diet to treat type 2 diabetes', *Nutr Metabol* 2: 34, doi:10.1186/1743-7075-2-34.

36 Office of Disease Prevention and Health Promotion (2015), *2015–2020 Dietary Guidelines for Americans*, health.gov/dietary guidelines/2015/.

37 Jane E. Brody (18 January 2016), 'What's new in the dietary guidelines', *New York Times*, well.blog.nytimes.com/2016/0/18 what's-new-in-the-dietary-guidelines/r_r=0.

38 L. Hooper et al. (September 2014), 'Reduced or modified dietary fat for preventing cardiovascular disease', *Cochrane DB Syst Rev*, doi: 10.1002/14651858.CD002137.

39 *Scientific Report of the 2015 Dietary Guidelines Advisory Committee* (2015), USDA & Department of Health and Human Services, Washington DC, p. 17, www.health.gov/dietaryguidelines/2015-scientific-report-PDFs/Scientific-Report-of-the-2015-Dietary-Guidelines-Advisory-Committee.pdf.

40 P. Whoriskey (18 December 2015), 'Congress: we need to review the dietary guidelines for Americans', *Washington Post*, www.washingtonpost.com/news/wonk/wp/2015/12/18/congress-we-need-to-review-the-dietary-guidelines-for-americans.

41 M.B. Schulze et al. (2004), 'Sugar-sweetened beverages, weight gain, and type 2 diabetes in young and middle-aged women', *JAMA* 292: 927–34.

42 InterAct Consortium (2013), 'Consumption of sweet beverages and type 2 diabetes incidence in European adults: results from EPIC-InterAct', *Diabetologia* 56: 1520–30.

43 S. Basu et al. (2013), 'The relationship of sugar to population-level diabetes prevalence: an econometric analysis of repeated cross-sectional data', *PLOS ONE* 8: e57873. Doi:10.1371/journal.pone.0057873.

44 T. Spector (2015), *The Diet Myth*, Weidenfeld and Nicolson, London, p. 4.

45 S. Basu et al. (2012), 'Nutritional determinants of worldwide diabetes: an econometric study of food markets and diabetes prevalence in 173 countries', *Pub Health Nutr*, doi: 10.1017/S1368980012002881.

46 M. Franco et al. (2007), 'Impact of energy intake, physical activity, and population-wide weight loss on cardiovascular disease and diabetes mortality in Cuba, 1980–2005', *Am J Epidemiol*, doi: 10.1093/aje/kwm226.

47 C. Gorry (2009), 'Cubans team up for better nutrition', *MEDICC Review* 11: 20–22; C. Porrata (2008), 'Cubans' deadly diet: a wake-up call', *MEDICC Review* 10: 52.

48 D. Cavan (2014), *Reverse Your Diabetes*, Vermilion, London.

49 N. Teicholz (2014), *The Big Fat Surprise*, Scribe, London, p. 46.

50 C.B. Ebbeling et al. (2012), 'Effects of dietary composition on energy expenditure during weight-loss maintenance', *JAMA* 307: 2627–34. See also B.M. Hron et al. (2015), 'Relationship of insulin dynamics to body composition and resting energy expenditure following weight loss', *Obesity (Silver Spring)* 23: 2216–22.

51 M.A. Cornier et al. (2005), 'Insulin sensitivity determines the effectiveness of dietary macronutrient composition on weight loss in obese women', *Obesity Res* 13: 703–9.

52 K.S.D. Kothapalli et al. (26 March 2016), 'Positive selection on a regulatory insertion-deletion polymorphism in FDDS2 influences apparent endogenous synthesis of arachidonic acid', *Mol Biol Evol*, doi: 10.1093/molbev/msw049.

16: The carbohydratisation of the English-speaking breakfast

1 C.H.S. Ruxton and T.R. Kirk (1997), 'Breakfast: a review of associations with measures of dietary intake, physiology and biochemistry', *Br J Nutr* 78: 199–213.

17: Nothing about breakfast makes sense except in the light of insulin

1 Adapted from Laios et al. (2012), 'Arataeus of Cappadocia and the first description of diabetes', *Hormones* 11: 109–13.

2 Described by R. Bilous and R. Donnelly (2010), *Handbook of Diabetes*, 4th edn, Wiley-Blackwell, Oxford, p. 6.

3 F.G. Banting, C.H. Best, J.B. Collip, W.R. Campbell and A.A. Fletcher (1922), 'Pancreatic extracts in the treatment of diabetes mellitus', *Can Med Assoc J* 12: 141–6.

4 Julian Wood (16 July 2010), 'Penicillin: the Oxford story', http://www.ox.ac.uk/media/science_blog/00716.html. Accessed 17 October 2014. Alexander made a wonderful initial recovery from his infection, but unfortunately the supplies of penicillin ran out and he died. Yet the next four patients to be treated made good – indeed, then-miraculous – recoveries.

5 American Diabetes Association (2014), 'Diagnosis and classification of diabetes mellitus: position statement', *Diabetes Care*, 37: S81–90.

6 Quoted in Richard Dods (2013), *Understanding Diabetes: A Biochemical Perspective*, John Wiley, New Jersey, pp. 27–8.

7 E.A.M. Gale (2001), 'The discovery of type 1 diabetes', *Diabetes* 50: 217–26.

8 Mark Daly et al. (1998), 'Acute effects on insulin sensitivity and diurnal metabolic profiles of a high-sucrose compared with a high starch diet', *Am J Clin Nutr* 67: 1186–96.

9 Shona Livingstone (6 January 2015), 'Estimated life expectancy in a Scottish cohort with type 1 diabetes, 2008–2010', *J Am Med Assoc*, doi: 10.1001/jama.2014.16425.

10 Quoted by Richard Dods (2013), *Understanding Diabetes: A Biochemical Perspective*, John Wiley, New Jersey, p. 323.

18: Diabesity, the big new disease

1 B. Caballero (2007), 'The global epidemic of obesity: An overview', *Epidemiol Rev* 29: 1–5, doi:10.1093/epirev/mxm012. PMID17569676.

2 World Health Organization (1995), 'Physical status: the use and interpretation of anthropometry', *WHO Technical Report Series 854*, http://whqlibdoc.who.int/trs/WHO_TRS_854.pdf.

3 G.A. Colditz et al. (1995), 'Weight gain as a risk factor for clinical diabetes in women', *Ann Intern Med* 122: 481–6.

4 Prospective Studies Collaboration (2009), 'Body-mass index and cause-specific mortality in 900,000 adults: collaborative analyses of 57 prospective studies', *Lancet* 373: 1083–96.

5 R.F. Hammann et al. (2006), 'Effect of weight loss with lifestyle intervention on risk of diabetes', *Diabetes Care* 29: 2102–7.

6 M. Ng, T. Fleming, M. Robinson, B. Thomson, N. Graetz, C. Margono et al. (2014), 'Global, regional, and national prevalence of overweight and obesity in children and adults during 1980–2013: a systematic analysis for the Global Burden of Disease Study 2013', *Lancet*, doi:10.1016/S0140-6736(14)60460-8. ISSN 0140-6736. These rates have been rising. In the USA, for example, obesity rates doubled between 1980 and 2002, while in the UK they tripled between 1980 and 2008/9.

7 C.L. Ogden et al. (2004), 'Mean body weight, height and body mass index, United States 1960–2002', *CDC Advance Data*, www.cdc/nchs/data/as347.pdf. Accessed 2 December 2015.

8 NCD Risk Factor Collaboration (2016), 'Trends in body-mass index in 200 countries from 1975 to 2014: a pooled analysis of 1698 population-based studies with 19.2 million participants', *Lancet* 387: 1377–96.

9 D.H. Bessesen (2008), 'Update on obesity', *J Clin Endocrinol Metab* 93: 2027–34, doi:10.1210/jc.2008-0520. PMID 18539769.

10 G. Swerling (29 December 2015), 'Thousands of obese people rescued from their own homes', *The Times*, p. 19.

11 OECD (2014), *Update on Obesity*, http://www.oecd.org/els/health-systems/Obesity-Update-2014.pdf.

12 G. Whitlock et al. (2009), 'Body-mass index and cause-specific mortality in 900,000 adults: collaborative analyses of 57 prospective studies', *Lancet* 373: 1083–96.

13 D.B. Allison, K.R. Fontaine, J.R. Manson, J. Stevens and T.B. Vanitallie (1999), 'Annual deaths attributable to obesity in the United States', *JAMA* 282: 1530–38, doi:10.1001/jama.282.16.1530. PMID 10546692.

14 Centers for Disease Control and Prevention (2010), 'Vital signs: state-specific obesity prevalence among adults – United States, 2009', *Morbid Mortal Weekly Report*, Vol. 59.

15 McKinsey Global Institute (2014), 'Overcoming obesity: an initial economic analysis', http://www.mckinsey.com/search.aspx?q=obesity+cost. Accessed 26 November 2014.

16 Eurostat (15 April 2016), 'Statistics explained: overweight and obesity – BMI_ statistics', see http://epp.eurostat.ec.europa.eu/statistics_explained/index.php/Overweight_and_obesity_–_BMI_statistics. Accessed 15 October 2016.

17 American Diabetes Association (1 April 2016), *National Diabetes Statistics Report*. See: http://www.diabetes.org/diabetes-basics/statistics/. Accessed 15 October 2016.

18 Centers for Disease Control and Prevention (April 2016), *Long Term Trends in Diabetes*, www.cdc.gov/diabetes/statistics/slides/long_term_trends/pdf. Accessed 4 August 2016.

19 American Diabetes Association (2013), 'Economic Costs of Diabetes in the U.S. in 2012', *Diabetes Care 36*: 1033–46.

20 Centers for Disease Control and Prevention (7 October 2016), *Deaths and Mortality*, www.cdc.gov/nchs/fastats/deaths.htm. Accessed 15 October 2016.

21 Diabetes UK (2014), *Statistics*. See http://www.diabetes.org.uk/ Accessed 15 October 2016. About_us/What-we-say/Statistics/Diabetes-prevalence-2013/. See also J. Woodfield (2016), 'Diabetes rates in UK hit four million for first time, new figures show', www.diabetes.co.uk/news/2016/jan/diabetes-rates-in-uk-hits-four-million-for-first-time,-new-figures-show-97453170.htmol. Accessed 8 January 2016.

22 Diabetes UK, *Reach for the Stars*, www.diabetes.org.uk/Documents/About%20Us/reach%20the%20Stars%20Strategy%20summary.pdf. Accessed 1 November 2014.

23 World Health Organization (May 2014), 'The top 10 causes of death', http://www.who.int/mediacentre/factsheets/fs310/en/.

24 International Diabetes Federation (2010), *Diabetes Facts*, www.idf.org.

25 B. Wansink and C.S. Wansink (2010), 'The largest last supper: depictions of portion size and plate size increased over the millennium', *Int J Obes*, 34: 943–4, doi:10.1038/ijo.2010.37.

26 The most accessible criticism of the Wansinks' study was provided by Bendor Grosvenor in the *Guardian* newspaper of Tuesday, 6 April 2010 in his article 'Last Supper paintings can't tell us much about trends in overeating', http://www.theguardian.com/commentisfree/2010/apr/06/last-supper-obesity-art-history. The art historian Sarah Rich made a scholarly criticism in her 'Reply to B. Wansink and C.S. Wansink' (2011), *Int J Obes* 35: 462.

27 Quoted by Reuters (23 March 2010), 'Super-Sizing the "Last Supper"', http://www.reuters.com/article/us-food-lastsupper-odd-id USTRE62M35U20100323.

28 Centers for Disease Control and Prevention (6 February 2004), 'Trends in intake of energy and macronutrients, United States, 1971–2000', *Morbid Mortal Weekly Report,* Vol. 53.

29 National Heart, Lung, and Blood Institute (13 February 2013), *Balance Food and Activity,* www.nhlbi.nih.gov/healtyh/educational/wecan/healthy-weight-basics/balance.htm.

30 R.J. Kuczmarski et al. (1994), 'Increasing prevalence of overweight among US adults', *JAMA* 272: 205–11.

31 Bureau of Labor Statistics (3 August 2006), '100 years of US consumer spending', www.bis.gov/opud/uscs/. Popularised by D. Thomson (5 April 2012), *Atlantic,* www.theatlantic.com/how-america- spends-money-100-years-in-the-life-of-the-family-budget/ 255475/.

32 S. Wiggins et al. (2015), *The Rising Cost of a Healthy Diet,* Overseas Development Institute, London.

33 C. Monteiro (2010), 'The big issue is ultra-processing', *World Nutr* 1: 237–69.

34 N.M. Avena, P. Rada and B.G. Hoebel (2009), 'Sugar and fat bingeing have notable differences in addictive-like behavior', *J Nutr* 139: 623–8.

35 M. Moss (2013), *Salt Sugar Fat: How the Food Giants Hooked Us,* Random House, New York.

36 Well illustrated in the *Google* entry for High fructose corn syrup. Accessed 8 April 2016.

37 http://www.pbs.org/wgbh/pages/frontline/shows/diet/themes/lowfat.html. Accessed 19 May 2016.

38 B.M. Popkin and K.J. Duffey (2010), 'Does hunger and satiety drive eating anymore? Increasing eating occasions and decreasing time between eating occasions in the United States', *Am J Clin Nutr* 91: 1342–7.

39 Dervla Murphy (1968), *In Ethiopia with a Mule*, John Murray, London, p. 43.

40 Y.N. Harari (2014), *Sapiens: A Brief History of Humankind*, Harvill Secker, London, pp. 388–9.

41 C. Griffiths and A. Brock (Summer 2003), 'Twentieth century mortality trends in England and Wales', *Health Stat Quart* 18: 4–17.

42 www.cooksinfo.com/british-wartime-food. Accessed November 2015.

43 N. Medic et al. (13 April 2016), 'The presence of real food usurps hypothetical health value judgement in overweight people', *eNeuro*, doi: 10.1523/NEURO.0025-16.2016; N. Medic et al. (22 March 2016), 'Increased body mass index is associated with specific regional alterations in brain structure', *Int J Obes*, doi: 10.1038/ijo.2016.42.

44 O. Bowcott (18 December 2014), 'Obesity can be a disability, EU court rules', *Guardian*, www.theguardian.com/society/2014/dec/18/obesity-can-be-disability-eu-court-rules.

45 S.E. Jackson et al. (2014), 'Perceived weight discrimination and changes in weight, waist circumference, and weight status', *Obesity* 22: 2485–8.

46 See among the many studies reporting on the denial by obese people: D. Lansky (1982), 'Estimates of food quantity and calories: errors in self-report among obese patients', *Am J Clin Nutr* 35: 727–32; M. Barbara et al. (2003), 'Markers of the validity of reported energy intake', *J Nutr* 133: 895S–920S; J.A. Tooze et al. (2004), 'Psychosocial predictors of energy underreporting in a large doubly labelled water study', *Am J Clin Nutr* 79: 795–804; F. Johnson et al. (2014), 'Do weight perceptions among obese adults in Great Britain match clinical definitions? Analysis of cross-sectional surveys from 2007 to 2012', *BMJ Open* 4: e005561.

47 J.A. Black et al. (2015), 'Child obesity cut-offs as derived from parental perceptions: cross-sectional questionnaire', *Br J Gen Pract*, doi:10.3399/bjgp15X68.

48 D.T. Duncan et al. (2015), 'Change in misconception of child's body weight among parents of American preschool children', *Childhood Obesity* 11: 384–93.

49 Chimamanda Ngozi Adiche (2013), *Americanah*, Fourth Estate, London, pp. 5–6.

50 Ross C. Brownson, Tegan K. Boehmer and Douglas A. Luke (2005), 'Declining rates of physical activity in the United States: what are the contributors?', *Ann Rev Pub Health* 26: 421–43. The findings in this study are similar to those seen in Europe and comparable continents such as Australasia.

51 L. Lanningham-Foster, L.J. Nysse and J.A. Levine (2003), 'Labor saved, calories lost: the energetic impact of domestic labor-saving devices', *Obes Res* 11: 1178–81.

52 W.L. Haskell (1996), 'Physical activity, sport, and health: toward the next century', *Res Q Exerc Sport* 67 (3, suppl): S37–47, quoted in W.G. Thompson et al. (2007), 'Treatment of obesity', *Mayo Clin Proc* 82: 93–102.

53 A.W. Barclay and J. Brand-Miller (2011), 'The Australian paradox: a substantial decline in sugar intake over the same timeframe that overweight and obesity have increased', *Nutrition* 3: 491–504.

54 M. Safi (20 July 2014), *Guardian*, www.theguardian.com/world/2014/jul/21/sugar-row-nutritionists-cleared-misconduct.

55 British Heart Foundation (2012), *Coronary Heart Disease Statistics 2012*, p. 124, www.bhf.org.uk/publications/statistics/coronary-heart-disease-statistics-2012.

56 House of Commons Health Committee, *Obesity: Third Report of Session 2003–04*, p. 24, www.publications.parliament.uk/pa/cm 200304/cmselect/cmhealth/23/23.pdf.

57 C.H.M. van Jaarsveld and M.C. Gulliford (2015), 'Childhood obesity trends from primary care electronic health records between 1994 and 2013: population-based cohort study', *Arch Dis Child* 2015: 1–6.

58 Nassim Taleb (2012), *Antifragile: Things That Gain from Disorder*, Random House, New York.

59 K.M. Flegal et al. (2005), 'Excess deaths associated with underweight, overweight, and obesity', *JAMA* 293: 1861–7.

60 M. Lenz et al. (2009), 'The morbidity and mortality associated with overweight and obesity in adulthood: a systematic review', *Dtsch Arztebl Int* 106: 641–8; H.M. Orpana et al. (2010), 'BMI and mortality: results from a national longitudinal study of Canadian adults', *Obesity (Silver Spring)* 18: 214–18.

61 V. Hughes (2013), 'The big fat truth', *Nature* 497: 428–30.

62 J. Miller (23 February 2013), 'Weight and mortality: Harvard researchers challenge results of obesity analysis', *Harvard Gazette*, News.harvard.edu/gazette/story/2013/02/weight-and-mortality/.

63 K.M. Flegal et al. (2013), 'Association of all-cause mortality with overweight and obesity using standard body mass index categories', *JAMA* 309: 71–82.

64 C.E. Hastie et al. (2010), 'Obesity paradox in a cohort of 4880 consecutive patients undergoing percutaneous coronary intervention', *Eur Heart J* 31: 222–6.

65 British Heart Foundation (8 June 2015), 'How fat can help fight heart disease', www.bhf.org.uk/news-from-the-bhf/news-archive/2015/june/ how-fat-can-help-fight-heart-disease. Accessed 4 July 2015.

66 The original report is in Danish and though it has a good summary in English it can be best accessed by Anglophones via C.P. Persson (2013), 'New report: weight loss increases mortality', *ScienceNordic*, sciencenordic.com/new-report-weight-loss-increases-mortality. Accessed 7 August 2015. Samuel Preston of Boston University takes a different perspective: reviewing 6,276 subjects, he found that the best predictor of people's mortality was their historical maximum weight (i.e. the heaviest you've ever been) and that weight loss disguises the fact that maximal-weight seems to cause irreparable damage (A. Stokes and S.H. Preston (2016), 'Revealing the burden of obesity using weight histories', *PNAS*, pnas.org/cgi/doi/0.1073/pnas.1515472113). But neither he nor the Danes could exclude the possibility that illness might cause people to lose weight, and so distort their interpretation of the data.

19: Insulin-resistance, the modern plague

1 H. John (1928), 'Diabetes: a statistical study of two thousand cases', *Arch Intern Med* 42: 217–47.

2 J. Bagdale, E. Bierman and D. Porte (1967), 'The significance of basal insulin levels in the evaluation of the insulin response to glucose in diabetic and nondiabetic subjects', *J Clin Invest* 46: 1549–57.

3 D.R. Matthews and P.C. Matthews (2010), 'Type 2 diabetes as an "infectious" disease: is this the Black Death of the 21st century?', *Diabetic Med* 28: 2–9.

4 S. Del Prato, F. Leonetti, D.C. Simonson et al. (1994), 'Effect of sustained physiologic hyperinsulinemia and hyperglycaemia on insulin secretion and insulin sensitivity in man', *Diabetologia* 37: 1025–35; P. Iozzo, T. Pratipanawatr, H. Pijl et al (2001), 'Physiological hyperinsulinemia impairs insulin-stimulated glycogen synthase activity and glycogen synthesis', *Am J Physiol* 280: E712–19.

5 R.C. Hermans et al. (2012), 'Mimicry of food intake: the dynamic interplay between eating companions', *PLOS One* 7(2), doi: 10.1371/journal.pone.0031027.

6 Barbara B. Kahn and Jeffrey S. Flier (2000), 'Obesity and insulin resistance', *J Clin Invest* 106: 473–81.

7 Diabetes UK (2009), *Prediabetes: Preventing the Type 2 Diabetes Epidemic*, http://www.diabetes.org.uk/ Documents/Reports/Pre diabetesPreventingthe Type2diabetesepidemic Oct2009report.pdf. The incidence is rising and, in 2010, 79 million Americans (35 per cent of the population) had it.

8 A.G. Mainous III, R.J. Tanner, R. Baker et al. (2014), 'Prevalence of prediabetes in England from 2003 to 2011: population-based,

cross-sectional study', *BMJ Open* 2014; 4: e005002. doi:10.1136/.

9 Y. Xu et al. (2013), 'Prevalence and control of diabetes in Chinese adults', *J Am Med Assoc* 310: 948–58.

10 The papers reporting that are listed in B.B. Lowell and G.I. Shulman (2005), 'Mitochondrial dysfunction and type 2 diabetes', *Science* 307: 384–7.

11 C.N. Hales and D.J.P. Barker (1992), 'Type 2 (non-insulin-dependent) diabetes mellitus: the thrifty phenotype hypothesis', *Diabetologia* 35: 595–601; C. Rhodes (2005), 'Type 2 diabetes – a matter of β-cell life and death?', *Science* 307: 380–84.

12 F.M. Ashcroft and P. Rorsman (2012), 'Diabetes mellitus and the β cell: the last ten years', *Cell* 148: 1160–71.

13 M. Straczkowski et al. (2003), 'Insulin resistance in the first-degree relatives of persons with type 2 diabetes', *Med Sci Monit* 9 CR: 186–90.

14 S. Kashyap et al. (2003), 'A sustained increase in plasma free fatty acids impairs insulin secretion in nondiabetic subjects genetically predisposed to develop type 2 diabetes', *Diabetes* 52: 2461–74.

15 R. Taylor and R.R. Holman (2015), 'Normal weight individuals who develop Type 2 diabetes: the personal fat threshold', *Clin Sci* 128: 405–10.

16 S. Steven et al. (2015), 'Weight loss decreases excess pancreatic triacylglycerol specifically in type 2 diabetes', *Diabetes Care*, doi: 10.2337/dc15-0750.

17 John E. Gerich (1998), 'The genetic basis of type 2 diabetes mellitus: impaired insulin secretion *versus* impaired insulin sensitivity', *Endocr Rev* 19: 491–503; S.E. Kahn (2003), 'The relative contributions of insulin resistance and beta-cell dysfunction to the pathophysiology of type 2 diabetes', *Diabetologia* 46: 3–19. As these two titles suggest, it's not always clear which defect – insulin-resistance or partial islet cell failure – comes first in each patient. This is because partial islet cell failure will lead to high levels of circulating blood glucose and of free fatty acids, and these – unexpectedly – will in turn lead to insulin-resistance: glucotoxicity and lipotoxicity can not only damage islets, they can also render the mass of cells glucose- and insulin-resistant. But these two papers confirm that, regardless of the initial genetic weakness, there is in type 2 diabetes a convergence on the same illness in the end.

20: Definitions

1 R. Bilous and R. Donnelly (2010), *Handbook of Diabetes*, 4th edn, Wiley-Blackwell, Oxford, p. 9.

2 Random blood glucose (mmol/l)	Plasma	Capillary	Whole
Diabetic	≥11.0	≥11.0	≥11.0

Fasting capillary blood glucose			
Normal	<6.1	<5.6	<5.6
Prediabetic	6.1–6.9	5.6–6.0	5.6–6.0
Diabetic	≥ 7.0	≥ 6.1	≥ 6.1

2-hour capillary blood glucose			
Normal	<7.8	<7.8	<6.7
Prediabetic	7.8–11.0	7.8–11.0	6.7–9.9
Diabetic	≥11.1	≥11.1	≥10.0

HbA1c
Normal
Prediabetic
Diabetic   ≥ 6.4 % (48 mmol/mol)

These figures come from the American Diabetes Association and the World Health Organization (as reported by Bilous and Donnelly, 2010, *Handbook of Diabetes*, 4th edn, Wiley-Blackwell, Oxford, p. 9).

3 NHS Diabetic Eye Screening Programme (2014), http://diabeticeye. screening.nhs.uk/statistics.

4 C. Bunce and R. Wormald (2008), 'Causes of blind certifications in England and Wales: April 1999–March 2000, *Eye* 22: 905–11. Though there is recent evidence that the intensive NHS screening for eye disease, and the improved glycaemic control of diabetics, are paying off, and that the incidence of diabetic blindness may be beginning to fall, relative to the incidence of inherited retinal diseases, which if confirmed will be wonderful news (G. Liew, M. Michaelides and C. Bunce (2014), 'A comparison of the causes of blindness certifications in England and Wales in working-age adults (16–64 years), 1999–2000 with 2009–2010', *BMJ Open* 2014; 4: e004015 doi:10.1136/bmjopen-2013-004015).

5 N.J. Morrish, S.L. Wang, L.K. Stevens et al. (2001), 'Mortality and causes of death in the WHO multinational study of vascular disease in diabetes', *Diabetologia* 44, suppl 2; s14–21.

6 National Diabetes Support Team (2006), *Diabetic Foot Guide*, www.diabetes.nhs.uk/document.php?o=219.

7 American Diabetes Association (2014), 'Diagnosis and classification of diabetes mellitus. Position statement', *Diabetes Care* 37: supplement 1, 581–90.

21: The dawn phenomenon

1 S. Panda, J.B. Hogenesch and S.A. Kay (2002), 'Circadian rhythms from flies to humans', *Nature* 417: 329–35.

2 A. Herxheimer and K.J. Petrie (2002, updated 2008), 'Melatonin for the prevention and treatment of jet lag', *Cochrane DB Syst Rev*, CD001520, doi: 10.1002/14651858.CD001520.

3 F. Chapotot et al. (1998), 'Cortisol secretion is related to electroencephalographic alertness in human subjects during daytime wakefulness', *J Clin Endocrinol Metab* 83: 4263–8.

4 Cortisol actually inhibits insulin action even at the level of muscles (D. Dimitriadis et al. (1997), 'Effects of glucocorticoid excess on the sensitivity of glucose transport and metabolism to insulin in rat skeletal muscle', *Biochem J* 321: 707–12), but it appears that the non-insulin uptake of glucose can compensate for that under the circumstances of fight and flight. This is sufficiently ill-understood that Macfarlane et al., in their review, wrote that 'These anti-insulin effects favour hyperglycaemia, putatively to fuel non-insulin-dependent glucose uptake and oxidation in the brain and active skeletal and cardiac muscle' (D.P. Macfarlane et al. (2008), 'Glucocorticoids and fatty acid metabolism in humans: fuelling fat redistribution in the metabolic syndrome', *J Endocrinol* 187: 189–204).

5 S.J. Gould and R. Lewontin (1979), 'The spandrels of San Marco and the Panglossian paradigm: a critique of the adaptationist programme', *Proc Roy Soc London B* 205: pp. 581–98.

6 R.W. McGilvery (1970), *Biochemistry* (2nd edn), Sanders, Philadelphia, PA, p. 694.

7 P. Schonfeld and G. Reiser (2013), 'Why does brain metabolism not favor burning of fatty acids to provide energy?', *J Cerebr Blood F Metabolism* 33: 1493–9.

8 M. Roden et al. (1996), 'Mechanism of free fatty acid-induced insulin resistance in humans', *J Clin Invest* 97: 2859–65; A. Jovanovic et al. (2009), 'The second-meal phenomenon in type 2 diabetes', *Diabetes Care* 32: 1199–201. It should be noted that C. Abraira and A.M. Lawrence (1978), in 'The Staub-Traugott phenomenon: effects of starvation', *Am J Clin Nutr* 31: 213–21, argue that the inhibition of insulin-mediated glucose uptake can be uncoupled from free fatty acids, but if so then, as Roden at al. argue, a closely related phenomenon must be involved, and the physiological effect will be the same.

9 T. Ruge et al. (2009), 'Fasted to fed trafficking of fatty acids in human adipose tissue reveals a novel regulatory step for enhanced fat storage', *J Clin Endocrinol Metab* 94: 1781–8.

22: The biochemists have been warning us for nearly a century that breakfast is dangerous

1 H. Staub (1921) and K. Traugott (1922), quoted by C. Abraira and A.M. Lawrence (1978), 'The Staub-Traugott phenomenon: effects of starvation', *Am J Clin Nutr* 31: 213–21.
2 A. Jovanovic et al. (2009), 'The second meal phenomenon is associated with enhanced muscle glycogen storage in humans', *Clin Sci* 117: 119–27.

23: My story, episode 2

1 J.T. Gonzalez et al. (2013), 'Breakfast and exercise contingently affect postprandial metabolism and energy balance in physically active males', *Br J Nutr* 110: 721–32.
2 H.P. Weingarten and D. Elston (1991), 'Food cravings in a college population', *Appetite* 17: 167–75.
3 C.K. Martin et al. (2011), 'Change in food cravings, food preferences, and appetite during a low-carbohydrate and low fat diet', *Obesity (Silver Spring)* 19: 1863–970.
4 T. Shiya et al. (2002), 'Plasma ghrelin levels in lean and obese humans and the effect of glucose on ghrelin secretion', *J Clin Endocrinol Metab* 87: 240–44.
5 E.A. Chowdhury et al. (2015), Carbohydrate-rich breakfast attenuates glycaemic, insulinaemic and ghrelin response to *ad libitum* lunch relative to morning fasting in lean adults', *Br J Nutr* 114: 98–107 (though it seems that breakfast actually enhances the ghrelin).
6 L.A. Panossian and S.C. Veasey (2012), 'Daytime sleepiness in obesity: mechanisms beyond obstructive sleep apnea – a review', *Sleep* 35: 605–15.
7 Diabetes.co.uk (2016), *Metabolic Syndrome*, www.diabetes.co.uk/diabetes-and-metabolic-syndrome.html. Accessed 26 March 2016.
8 F.A.J.L. Scheer, C.J. Morris and S.A. Shea (2013), 'The internal circadian clock increases hunger and appetite in the evening independent of food intake and other behaviours', *Obesity (Silver Spring)* 21: 421–3.
9 T. Parkner, J.K. Nielsen, T.D. Sandahl, B.M. Bibby, B.S. Jensen and J.S. Christiansen (2011), 'Do all patients with type 2 diabetes need breakfast?', *Eur J Clin Nutr* 65: 761–3.
10 David Zinczenko (2013), *The 8-Hour Diet*, Rodale, NY, pp. xvii–xix, 51.
11 James A. Betts et al. (2014), 'The causal role of breakfast in energy

balance and health: a randomized controlled trial in lean adults',
Am J Clin Nutr 100: 539–47.

12 Dr Betts trusts that the spontaneous casual exercise of breakfast
eaters may be healthful because: 'increasing activity is one of the
most important ways to improve health' (*University of Bath News*,
13 February 2016, 'Eating breakfast could help obese people get
more active', www.bath.ac.uk/news/2016/02/13/science-eating-
breakfast/. Accessed 19 March 2016) but breakfast increases blood
glucose levels, and since all raised levels of blood glucose are
dangerous, the price the breakfast eater pays in higher blood levels
of glucose may be greater than the benefits they derive from the
extra exercise. Indeed, as Dr Betts – who himself skips breakfast –
has suggested, there is nothing to stop a breakfast skipper from
taking formal morning exercise in the form of a run or swim or cycle
ride. They would thus enjoy the health benefits of exercise without
the disbenefits of post-breakfast blood glucose elevation.

24: What a modern plague looks like: the metabolic syndrome

1 G.M. Reaven (1988), 'Role of insulin resistance in human disease',
Diabetes 37: 1595.

2 G. Reaven et al. (2000), *Syndrome X – Overcoming the Silent Killer
that Can Give You a Heart Attack*, Simon & Schuster, New York.

3 Earl S. Ford (2005), 'Prevalence of the metabolic syndrome defined
by the International Diabetes Federation among adults in the US',
Diabetes Care 28: 2745–9.

4 R. Weiss et al. (2013), 'What is metabolic syndrome, and why are
children getting it?', *Ann N Y Acad Sci* 1281: 123–40. See references
11 and 48, 49 and 50.

5 A.H. Berg and P. Scherer (2005), 'Adipose tissue, inflammation, and
cardiovascular disease', *Circ Res* 96: 939–49.

6 J.-P. Despre and Isabelle Lemieux (2006), 'Abdominal obesity and
metabolic syndrome', *Nature* 444: 881–7.

7 M. Giuseppe et al. (2013), 'ESH/ESC guidelines for the management
of arterial hypertension', *Eur Heart J* 34: 2159–219.

8 D. Lloyd-Jones et al. (2010), 'Heart disease and stroke statistics
– 2010 update: a report from the American Heart Association',
Circulation 121: e46–215.

9 P. Singer et al. (1985), 'Postprandial hypertension in patients with
mild essential hypertension', *Hypertension* 7: 182–6; Ele Ferrannini
et al. (1997), 'Insulin resistance, hyperinsulinemia, and blood
pressure: role of age and obesity', *Hypertension* 30: 1144–9.

10 H.E. Botker and A. Moller (2013), 'OH NO – The continuing story

of nitric oxide, diabetes, and cardiovascular disease', *Diabetes* 62: 2645–7.

11 M.-S. Zhou et al. (2014), 'Link between insulin resistance and hypertension: what is the evidence from evolutionary biology?', *Diabetology & Metabolic Syndrome* 6, doi:10.1186/1758-5996-6-12.

12 A.H. Berg and P. Scherer (2005), 'Adipose tissue, inflammation, and cardiovascular disease', *Circ Res* 96: 939–49.

13 G.H. Goossens et al. (2006), 'Angiotensin II: a major regulator of subcutaneous adipose tissue blood flow in humans', *J Physiol* 571.2: 451–60.

14 P. Trayhurn (2014), 'Hypoxia and adipocyte physiology – implications for adipose tissue dysfunction in obesity', *Ann Rev Nutr* 34: 207–36.

15 J.A. Ryle and W.T. Russell (1949), 'The natural history of coronary disease. A clinical and epidemiological study', *Brit Heart J* 11: 370–89.

16 W. Kannel et al. (1961), 'Factors of risk in the development of heart disease – six years follow up experience. The Framingham study', *Ann Intern Med* 55: 33–50.

17 CDC (2011), 'Vital signs: prevalence, treatment and control of high levels of low-density lipoprotein cholesterol', *Morbid Mortal Weekly Report* 60: 109–14.

18 E.V. Kuklina, P. Yoon and J.N.L. Keenan (2009), 'Trends in high levels of low-density lipoprotein cholesterol in the United States, 1999–2006', *JAMA* 302: 2104–10.

19 U. Schwab et al. (2014), 'Effect of the amount and type of dietary fat on cardiometabolic risk factors and developing type-2 diabetes, cardiovascular disease, and cancer: a systematic review', *Food Nutr Res* 58: 25145, http://dx.doi.org/10.3402/fnr.v58.25145.

20 Martin Adiels et al. (2008), 'Overproduction of very low-density lipoproteins is the hallmark of the dyslipidaemia in the metabolic syndrome', *Arterioscler Thromb Vasc Biol* 28: 1225–36.

21 B.M. Volk (21 November 2014), 'Effects of step-wise increases in dietary carbohydrate on circulating saturated fatty acids and palmitoleic acid in adults with metabolic syndrome', *PLOS One*, doi: 10.1371/journal.pone.0113605.

22 S.M. Haffner et al. (1990), 'Cardiovascular risk factors in confirmed prediabetic individuals. Does the clock for coronary heart disease start ticking before the onset of clinical diabetes?', *JAMA* 263: 2893–8.

23 Frank B. Hu et al. (2002), 'Elevated risk of cardiovascular disease prior to clinical diagnosis of type 2 diabetes', *Diabetes Care* 25: 1129–34.

24 S.P. Weisberg et al. (2003), 'Obesity is associated with macrophage accumulation in adipose tissue', *J Clin Invest* 112: 1796–808.

25 A.H. Berg and P. Scherer (2005), 'Adipose tissue, inflammation, and cardiovascular disease', *Circ Res* 96: 939–49.

26 M. Ozata et al. (1999), 'Human leptin deficiency caused by a missense mutation: multiple endocrine defects, decreased sympathetic tone, and immune system dysfunction indicate new targets for leptin action, greater central than peripheral resistance to the effects of leptin, and spontaneous correction of leptin-mediated defects', *J Clin Endocrinol Metab* 84: 3686–95.

27 G. Matarese et al. (2005), 'Leptin in immunology', *J Immunol* 173: 3137–42; G. Paz-Filho et al. (2012), 'Leptin: molecular mechanisms, systematic pro-inflammatory effects, and clinical implications', *Arq Bras Endocrinol* 56: 597–607.

28 N. Ouchi and K. Walsh (2007), 'Adiponectin as an anti-inflammatory factor', *Clin Chem Acta* 380: 24–30.

29 P. Calder, G. Dimitriadis and P. Newsholme (2007), 'Glucose metabolism in lymphoid and inflammatory cells and tissues', *Curr Opin Clin Nutr* 10: 531–40. Roy Taylor has shown how the insulin receptor activities of immune and fat cells are unrelated, thus indicating how insulin-resistance of fat cells could direct glucose to immune cells (R. Taylor et al. (1984), 'The relationship between human adipocyte and monocyte insulin binding', *Clin Sci* 67: 139–42). Potentially, a similar uncoupling of liver and muscle cell insulin binding from inflammatory cell binding could direct glucose to inflammatory cells.

30 A.H. Berg and P. Scherer (2005), 'Adipose tissue, inflammation, and cardiovascular disease', *Circ Res* 96: 939–49.

31 E. Raynaud et al. (2000), 'Relationships between fibrinogen and insulin resistance', *Atherosclerosis* 150: 365–70; M.C. Alessi et al. (1997), 'Production of plasminogen activator inhibitor 1 by human adipose tissue: possible link between visceral fat accumulation and vascular disease', *Diabetes* 46: 860–67.

32 A. Martin, S. Normad, M. Sothier, J. Pyrat, C. Louche-Pelissier and M. Laville (2000), 'Is advice for breakfast consumption justified? Results from a short-term dietary and metabolic experiment in young healthy men', *Brit J Nutr* 84: 337–44.

33 James A. Betts et al. (2014), 'The causal role of breakfast in energy balance and health: a randomized controlled trial in lean adults', *Am J Clin Nutr* 100: 539–47.

34 E.A. Chowdhury et al. (10 February 2016), 'The causal role of breakfast in energy balance and health: a randomized controlled trial in obese people', *Am J Clin Nutr*, doi: 10.3945/ajcn.115.122044.

25: Can we reverse the metabolic syndrome?

1 Diabetes UK (2009), *Prediabetes: Preventing the Type 2 Diabetes Epidemic*, http://www.diabetes.org.uk/Documents/Reports/Pre diabetesPreventingtheType2 diabetesepidemicOct2009report.pdf.

2 Quoted in E. John (19 September 2010), 'Why exercise won't make you thin', *Observer*, www.theguardian.com/lifeandstyle/2010/sep/19/exercise-dieting-public-health.

3 Ibid.

4 L.R. Pedersen et al. (2015), 'A randomised trial comparing weight loss with aerobic exercise in overweight individuals with coronary heart disease: the CUT-IT trial', *Eur J Prev Cardiol* 22: 1009–17.

5 A.E. Fremeaux et al. (2011), 'The impact of school-time activity on total physical activity: the activistat hypothesis', *Int J Obes (Lond)* 35: 1277–83.

6 Quoted by E. John (19 September 2010), *Observer*, www.the guardian.com/lifeandstyle/2010/sep/19/exercise-dieting-public-health.

7 S. Bhutani et al. (2013), 'Alternative day fasting and endurance exercise combine to reduce body weight and favorably alter plasma lipids in obese humans', *Obesity* 21: 1370–79.

8 E.J. Henriksen (2002), 'Effects of acute exercise and exercise training on insulin resistance', *J Appl Physiol* 93: 788–96.

9 Diabetes Prevention Program Research Group (2002), 'Reduction in the incidence of type 2 diabetes with lifestyle intervention or metformin', *N Engl J Med* 346: 393–403.

10 O. Ekelund et al. (2015), 'Physical activity and all-cause mortality across levels of overall and abdominal obesity in European men and women: The European Prospective Investigation into Cancer and Nutrition Study (EPIC), *Am J Clin Nutr* 101: 1–9.

11 James Gallagher (15 January 2015), 'Inactivity "kills more than obesity"', *BBC News: Health*, www.bbc.co.uk/news/health-30812439. Accessed 15 January 2015.

12 G. Hogstrom et al. (2015), 'Aerobic fitness in late adolescence and the risk of early death: a prospective cohort study of 1.3 million Swedish men', *Int J Epidemiol*, doi: 10.1093/ije/dyv32.

13 V.B. O'Leary et al. (2006), 'Exercise-induced reversal of insulin resistance in obese elderly is associated with reduced visceral fat', *J Appl Physiol* 100: 1584–9.

14 S. Bailey, Foreword, in Academy of Medical Royal Colleges (2015), *Exercise: The Miracle Cure and the Role of the Doctor in Promoting It*, Academy of Medical Royal Colleges, London, p. 2, www.aomrc.org.uk/doc_download/9821-exercise-the-miracle-cure.

15 L. Dostalova et al. (2007), 'Increased insulin sensitivity in patients with anorexia nervosa: the role of adipocytokines', *Physiol Res* 56: 587–94.

16 S. Steven et al. (2016), 'Very-low-calorie diet and 6 months of weight stability in type 2 diabetes: pathophysiological changes in responders and nonresponders', *Diabetes Care*, doi: 10.23337/dc15-1942.

17 Drs Ferranni and Mingrone from Pisa, Italy, have reviewed the collective experience of reversing type 2 diabetes, and they concluded that, just by eating less, a patient's insulin levels will fall, so their insulin-resistance will start to reverse, so their insulin levels will further fall in a virtuous cycle (E. Ferranni and G. Mingrone (2009), 'Impact of different bariatric surgical procedures on insulin action and cell function in type 2 diabetes', *Diabetes Care* 32: 514–20). Other virtuous cycles are activated by weight loss: obesity causes inflammation, and inflammation provokes insulin-resistance and damages the islets of Langerhans, but in the words of a comprehensive review from the Albert Einstein College of Medicine, Bronx, NY, 'Weight loss decreases systematic inflammation' (A.H. Berg and P. Scherer (2005), 'Adipose tissue, inflammation, and cardiovascular disease', *Circ Res* 96: 939–49). Further, once a patient starts to lose weight, and once their raised levels of blood glucose and free fatty acids start to fall, the glucotoxicity and lipotoxicity of type 2 are alleviated and the islets can begin to recover.

And they *can* recover: the beta cells in the islets have a short lifespan of only about sixty days (they are constantly being replenished by new cells budding from the old ones or budding from other nearby pancreatic cells), so if a new generation of beta cells is born into a less hostile environment, they will do their jobs better, so their environment will improve, and they will enter into a virtuous cycle whereby improvements in the disease build on improvement (C.J. Rhodes (2005), 'Type 2 diabetes – a matter of α-cell life and death?', *Science* 307: 380–84).

18 Gastric bands are rings named on the American model of a wedding band. Thus gastric bands are silicone rings that wrap around the upper part of the stomach and so narrow it. On eating, therefore, the upper part of the patient's stomach fills up quickly, so they eat less. Bypass operations are more dramatic: a small part of the upper stomach is cut away and connected directly to the small intestine some distance 'downstream' from the usual exit of the stomach into the small intestine. Most of the stomach and some of the small intestine are thus bypassed, which means that, on eating, the upper part of the patient's stomach fills up quickly, so they eat less. The

food that is eaten, moreover, may be less well digested. In a sleeve gastrectomy, some two-thirds of the stomach is simply removed.

19 W.J. Pories, M.S. Swanson, K.G. MacDonald, S.B. Long, P.G. Morris, B.M. Brown, H.A. Barakat, R.A. deRamon, G. Israel and J.M. Dolezal (1995), 'Who would have thought it? An operation proves to be the most effective therapy for adult-onset diabetes mellitus', *Ann Surg* 222: 339–50.

20 The Mayo Clinic (2016), 'Type 2 Diabetes', http://www.mayoclinic.org/diseases-conditions/type-2-diabetes/symptoms-causes/dxc-20169861. Accessed 15 October 2016.

21 James Vaupel (2010), 'Biodemography of human ageing', *Nature* 464: 536–42.

22 I suspect that insulin-resistance per se is actually a feature of ageing. It has long been recognised that the numbers of receptors for a large number of hormones, including insulin, fall with age (G.S. Roth (1979), 'Hormone receptor changes during adulthood and senescence: significance for aging research', *Fed Proc* 38: 1910–14). So a fall in the numbers of insulin receptors on ageing may induce resistance to the hormone's actions. At any moment, though, we use only a small proportion of our insulin receptors, so we probably have the spare capacity to compensate for a fall in the number of receptors on ageing. Yet insulin-resistance per se may still emerge as a feature of ageing because there are molecular events downstream of the receptor that appear to decline on ageing. So a study on people aged 21–87 years old, performed by a research group from the Mayo Clinic itself, confirmed that though exercise could reverse many aspects of insulin-resistance in older people, nonetheless exercise could not reverse *all* of them (K.R. Short et al. (2003), 'Impact of aerobic exercise training on age-related changes in insulin sensitivity and muscle oxidative capacity', *Diabetes* 52: 1888–96). Yet a separate study from Naples, Italy, has shown that centenarians (people aged 100+) are extremely insulin-sensitive, which confirms that insulin-resistance is not an inevitable feature of ageing, and which also confirms that insulin-sensitivity is associated with longevity – and vice versa (M. Barbieri et al. (2001), 'Age-related insulin resistance: is it an obligatory finding? The lesson from healthy centenarians', *Diabetes Metab Res Rev* 17: 19–26). So the overall message is indeed that the current epidemic of type 2 diabetes is largely caused by overeating and by physical inactivity, but that ageing per se may also be a contributory factor.

23 M. Barbieri et al. (2001), 'Age-related insulin resistance: is it an obligatory finding? The lesson from healthy centenarians', *Diabetes Metab Res Rev* 17: 19–26.

24 H. Farin et al. (2006), 'Body mass index and waist circumference both contribute to differences in insulin-mediated glucose disposal in non-diabetic adults', *Am J Clin Nutr* 83: 47–51.

26: The new fasting diets

1 A. Freer (2015), *Eat. Nourish. Glow.*, Thorsons, HarperCollins, New York and London, pp. 112–13.

2 K. Varady, B. Gottlieb (2014), *The Every Other Day Diet* (UK edn), Yellow Kite, London, p. 1. (US edition 2013, Hachette.) For a more formal report from Dr Varady, please see A.R. Barnosky et al. (2014), 'Intermittent fasting vs daily calorie restriction for type 2 diabetes prevention: a review of human findings', *Transl Res* 164: 302–11.

3 C.M. Clay, Mary F. Crowell and L.A. Maynard (1935), 'The effect of retarded growth upon the length of the life span and upon the ultimate body size', *J Nutr* 10: 63–79.

4 See the references in Leanne M. Redman and Eric Ravussin (2011), 'Caloric restriction in humans: impact on physiological, psychological and behavioral outcomes', *Antioxid Redox Sign* 14: 275–87.

5 Ibid.

6 Anthony Civitarese et al. (March 2007), 'Calorie restriction increases muscle mitochondrial biogenesis in healthy humans', *PLOS One* 4 e76. The structures that generate the free radicals – the intracellular organelles known as mitochondria – are refreshed by caloric restriction, and when Dr Anthony Civitarese and his colleagues in Baton Rouge, Louisiana, reduced the food intake of thirty-six young overweight adults by 25 per cent over six months, their numbers of mitochondria rose by 35 per cent. But the new mitochondria seemed to be more efficient than the older ones, and Dr Civitarese speculated that in consequence their rate of free radical production fell.

7 M.V. Chakravarthy and F.W. Booth (2004), 'Eating, exercise, and "thrifty" genotypes: connecting the dots toward an evolutionary understanding of modern chronic diseases', *J Appl Physiol* 96: 3–10.

8 See the references and discussion in H. Sherman et al. (2012), 'Long-term restricted feeding alters circadian expression and reduces the level of inflammatory and disease markers', *J Cell Mol Med* 15: 2745–59.

9 S. Brandhorst et al. (2015), 'A periodic diet that mimics fasting promotes multi-system regeneration, enhances cognitive performance and healthspan', *Cell Metab* 22: 86–99.

10 A.R. Barnosky et al. (2014), 'Intermittent fasting vs daily calorie restriction for type 2 diabetes prevention: a review of human findings', *Transl Res* 164: 302–11.

11 M. Headland et al. (2016), 'Weight-loss outcomes: a systematic review and meta-analysis of intermittent energy restriction trials lasting a minimum of 6 months', *Nutrients* 8: 354, doi:10.3390/nu8060354.

12 K. Varady and B. Gottlieb (2014), *The Every Other Day Diet* (UK edn), Yellow Kite, London, p. 26. (US edition 2013, Hachette.)

13 J. Rothschild et al. (2014), 'Time-restricted feeding and risk of metabolic disease: a review of human and animal studies', *Nutr Rev* 72: 308–18.

14 David Zinczenko (2013), *The 8-Hour Diet*, Rodale, NY, p. 15.

15 M. Hatori et al. (2012), 'Time-restricted feeding without reducing caloric intake prevents metabolic diseases in mice fed a high-fat diet', *Cell Metab* 15: 848–60.

16 K.-A. Stokkan et al. (2001), 'Entrainment of the circadian clock in the liver by feeding', *Science* 291: 490–93.

17 O. Froy (2012), 'Circadian rhythms and obesity in mammals', *International Scholarly Research Network: ISRN Obesity*, Article ID 437198, doi:10.5402/2012/437198.

18 M. Hatori and S. Panda (2010), 'CRY links the circadian clock and CREB-mediated gluconeogenesis', *Cell Res* 20: 1285–8.

19 S. Panda et al. (2002), 'Coordinated transcription of key pathways in the mouse by the circadian clock', *Cell* 109: 307–20.

20 David Zinczenko (2013), *The 8-Hour Diet*, Rodale, NY, pp. 19–20.

21 H. Sherman et al. (2012), 'Long-term restricted feeding alters circadian expression and reduces the level of inflammatory and disease markers', *J Cell Mol Med* 15: 2745–59.

22 H. Sherman et al. (2012), 'Timed high-fat diet resets circadian metabolism and prevents obesity', *FASEB J* 26: 3493–502.

23 H. Kahleova et al. (2014), 'Eating two larger meals a day (breakfast and lunch) is more effective than six smaller meals in a reduced-energy regimen for patients with type 2 diabetes: a randomised crossover study', *Diabetologia*, doi 10.1007/s00125-014-3253-5.

24 R.R. Henry et al. (1993), 'Intensive conventional insulin therapy for type I diabetes: metabolic effects during a 6 month outpatient trial', *Diabetes Care* 16: 21–31.

25 T.J. Horton et al. (1995), 'Fat and carbohydrate overfeeding in humans: different effects on energy storage', *Am J Clin Nutr* 62: 19–29; K.D. Hall et al. (2015), 'Calorie for calorie, dietary fat restriction results in more body fat loss than carbohydrate restriction in people with obesity', *Cell Metab* 22: 427–36.

26 C.K. Martin et al. (2011), 'Change in food cravings, food preferences, and appetite during a low-carbohydrate and low-fat diet', *Obesity (Silver Spring)* 19: 1963–70.

27 O. Carlson et al. (2007), 'Impact of reduced meal frequency without caloric restriction on glucose regulation in healthy, normal weight middle-aged men and women', *Metabolism* 56: 1729–34.

28 David Zinczenko (2013), *The 8-Hour Diet*, Rodale, NY, p. 36.

29 A. Roberts (2014), *Napoleon the Great*, Allen Lane, London, pp. 24, 790–91.

30 David Zinczenko (2013), *The 8-Hour Diet*, Rodale, NY, pp. xvii–xix, 51.

27: Type 3 diabetes (and other consequences of the metabolic syndrome)

1 R.A. DeFronzo (2010), 'Insulin resistance, lipotoxicity, type 2 diabetes and atherosclerosis: the missing links', *Diabetalogia* 53: 1270–87.

2 Ibid.

3 S.M. de la Monte and M. Tong (2014), 'Brain metabolic dysfunction at the core of Alzheimer's disease', *Biochem Pharmacol* 88: 548–59.

4 British Heart Foundation (2011), *Trends in Coronary Heart Disease 1961–2011*, http://www.bhf.org.uk/publications/view-publication. aspx?ps=1001933.

5 C.N. Hales and D.J.P. Barker (1992), 'Type 2 (non-insulin-dependent) diabetes mellitus: the thrifty phenotype hypothesis', *Diabetologia* 35: 595–610.

6 R. Weindruch and R.S. Sohal (1997), 'Caloric intake and aging', *N Eng J Med* 337: 986–94.

7 P.L. Hofman et al. (1997), 'Insulin resistance in short children with intrauterine growth retardation', *J Clin Endocr Metab* 82: 402–6.

8 A. Akesson et al. (2014), 'Low-risk diet and lifestyle habits in the primary prevention of myocardial infarction in men', *J Am Coll Cardiol* 64: 1299–306.

9 T.T. Fung et al. (2005), 'Diet-quality scores and plasma concentrations of markers of inflammation and endothelial dysfunction', *Am J Clin Nutr* 82: 163–73.

10 K. Lay (23 September 2014), 'Eight out of ten heart attacks prevented by healthier living', *The Times*, p. 21.

11 C.P. Nelson et al. (2015), 'Genetically determined height and coronary heart disease', *New Engl J Med*, doi:10.1056/NEJM 1404881.

12 J. Green et al. (2011), 'Height and cancer incidence in the Million Women Study: prospective cohort, and meta-analysis of prospective studies of height and total cancer risk', *Lancet Oncol* 12: 785–94.

13 A. Goggins and G. Matten (2016), *The Sirtfood Diet: The*

Revolutionary Plan for Health and Weight Loss, Yellow Kite, London.

14 K. Pallauff et al. (2013), 'Nutrition and healthy ageing: calorie restriction or polyphenol-rich "MediterrAsian" diet?', *Oxid Med Cel Longev*, http://dx.doi.org/10.1155/2013/707421.

15 C. Burnett et al. (2011), 'Absence of effects of Sir2 overexpression on lifespan in C elegans and Drosophila', *Nature* 477: 482–5.

16 M. Rivalland (2 January 2016), 'I lost almost half a stone', *The Times* magazine, p. 25.

17 L. Wilhelmsen et al. (2015), 'Men born in 1913 followed to age 100 years', *Scand Cardiovas J* 48: 45–8.

18 P.J. van Diest, et al. (1998), 'Pathology of silicone leakage from breast implants', *J Clin Pathol* 51: 493–7.

19 N.J. Morrish, S.L. Wang, L.K. Stevens, J.H. Fuller and H. Keen (2001), 'Mortality and causes of death in the WHO Multinational Study of Vascular Disease in Diabetes', *Diabetalogia* 44: S14–21.

20 X. Wang et al. (2013), 'Cholesterol levels and risk of hemorrhagic stroke: a systematic review and meta-analysis', *Stroke* 44: 21833–9.

21 M. Rauchhaus et al. (2003), 'The relationship between cholesterol and survival in patients with chronic heart failure', *J Am Coll Cardiol* 42: 1933–40.

22 Y. Homma et al. (2010), 'Effects of low-dose simvastatin on the distribution of plasma cholesterol and oxidised low-density lipoprotein in three ultra-centrifugally separated low-density lipoprotein subfractions: 12-month open-label trial', *J Athero Throm* 17: 1049–53.

23 Alexios Antonopolous et al. (2012), 'Statins as anti-inflammatory agents in atherogenesis: molecular mechanisms and lessons from recent clinical trials', *Curr Pharma Design* 18: 1519–30.

24 M.J. Pencina et al. (2014), 'Application of new cholesterol guidelines to a population-based sample', *N Engl J Med* 370: 1422–31.

25 Michelle Roberts (12 February 2014), 'Guidelines call for more people to be put on statins', *BBC News*, www.bbc.co.uk/news/health-26132758.

26 John Abramson (19 March 2015), 'Prescribing statins: time to rein it in', *Pharmaceut J* 284, doi:10.1211/PJ2015.20068145.

27 Chun-Xiao Xu, Hong-Hong Zhu and Yi-Min Zhu (2014), 'Diabetes and cancer: associations, mechanisms, and implications for medical practice', *World J Diabet* 5: 372–80.

28 Hans-Werner Hense, Hiltraud Kajüter, Jürgen Wellmann and Wolf U. Batzler (2011), 'Cancer incidence in type 2 diabetes patients – first results from a feasibility study of the D2C cohort', *Diabetology & Metabolic Syndrome* 3: 15, doi:10.1186/1758-5996-3-15.

29 Edward Giovannucci et al. (2010), 'Diabetes and cancer: a consensus report', *Diabetes Care* 33: 1674–85, doi: 10.2337/dc10-0666.

30 Alzheimer's Association (2010), 'Alzheimer's disease facts and figures', *Alzheimers Dement* 6: 158–94, doi: 10.1016/j.jalz.2010. 01.009.

31 C.L. Satizabal et al. (2016), 'Incidence of dementia over three decades in the Framingham heart study', *N Engl J Med* 374: 523–32.

32 The Mayo Clinic (17 June 2014), 'Alzheimer's disease', http://www. mayoclinic.org/diseases-conditions/alzheimers-disease/basics/.

33 Alzheimer's Association (2010), 'Alzheimer's disease facts and figures', *Alzheimers Dement* 6: 158–94, doi: 10.1016/j.jalz.2010.01.009.

34 F.G. De Felice and S.T. Ferreira (2014), 'Inflammation, defective insulin signaling, and mitochondrial dysfunction as common molecular denominators connecting type 2 diabetes to Alzheimer disease', *Diabetes* 63: 2262–72.

35 Alzheimer's Association of America (2015), 'Diabetes and cognitive decline', https://www.alz.org/national/documents/topicsheet_ diabetes.pdf. Accessed 15 October 2016.

36 A. Ott et al. (1999), 'Diabetes mellitus and the risk of dementia: the Rotterdam study', *Neurology* 53: 1937–42.

37 P.K. Crane et al. (2013), 'Glucose levels and risk of dementia', *N Engl J Med* 369: 540–48.

38 Cristina Carvalho, Paige S. Katz, Somhrita Dutta, Prasad V.G. Katakam, Paula I. Moreira and David W. Busija (2013), 'Increased susceptibility to amyloid-X toxicity in rat brain microvascular endothelial cells under hyperglycemic conditions', *J Alzheimers Dis* 38: 75–83.

39 N. Vagelatos and G. Eslick (2013), 'Type 2 diabetes as a risk factor for Alzheimer's disease: a meta-analysis and systematic review of the confounders, interactions and neuropathology associated with this relationship', *Alzheimers Dement* 9: Supplement, 136–7.

40 D. Kapogiannis et al. (23 October 2014), 'Dysfunctionally phosphorylated type 1 insulin receptor substrate in neural-derived blood exosomes of preclinical Alzheimer's disease', *FASEB J*, doi:10. 1096/fj.

41 National Institutes of Health (2000), *Preventing Alzheimer's Disease and Cognitive Decline*, http://consensus.nih.gov/2010/alzstatement.htm.

42 T. Ngandu et al. (2015), 'A 2 year multidomain intervention of diet, exercise, cognitive training and vascular risk monitoring versus control to prevent cognitive decline in at-risk elderly people (FINGER): a randomised controlled trial', *Lancet*, http://dx.doi.org/ 10.1016/S0140-6736(15)60461-5.

43 N. Qizilbash et al. (2015), 'BMI and risk of dementia in two million

people over two decades: a retrospective cohort study', *Lancet Diabet Endocrinol*, http://dx.doi.org/10.1016/S2213-8587(15)00033-9.

44 Y.-F. Chuang et al. (1 September 2015), 'Midlife adiposity predicts earlier onset of Alzheimer's dementia, neuropathology and presymptomatic cerebral amyloid accumulation', *Mol Psyc*, doi:10. 1038/mp.2015.129.

45 C.J. Steves et al. (2015), 'Kicking back cognitive ageing: leg power predicts cognitive ageing after ten years in older female twins', *Gerontology*, doi:10.1159/0004411029.

46 J.L. Cummings et al. (2014), 'Alzheimer's disease drug-development pipeline: few candidates, frequent failures', *Alzheimers Res Ther* 6: 37, http://alzres.com/content/6/4/37

28: So, what to eat?

1 L. Azadbakht and A. Esmaillzadeh (2009), 'Red meat intake associated with metabolic syndrome and the plasma C-reactive protein concentration in women', *J Nutr* 139: 335–9.

2 J. Barbaresko et al. (2013), 'Dietary pattern analysis and biomarkers of low-grade inflammation: a systematic literature review', *Nutr Rev* 71: 511–27.

3 F.M. Sacks et al. (1985), 'Plasma lipoprotein levels in vegetarians: the effect of ingestion of fats from dairy products', *JAMA* 254: 1337–41.

4 D. Ornish et al. (1990), 'Can lifestyle changes reverse coronary heart disease? The Lifestyle Heart Trial', *Lancet* 336: 129–33.

5 N.D. Bernard et al. (2006), 'A low-fat vegan diet improves glycemic control and cardiovascular risk factors in a randomized clinical trial in individuals with type 2 diabetes', *Diabetes Care* 29: 1777–83.

6 R. Sinha et al. (2009), 'Meat intake and mortality: a prospective study of over half a million people', *Arch Int Med* 169: 562–71; A. Pan et al. (2012), 'Red meat consumption and mortality: results from two prospective cohort studies', *Arch Int Med* 172: 555–63; S. Rohrman et al. (2013), 'Meat consumption and mortality – results from the European Prospective Investigation in cancer and nutrition', *BMC Medicine* 11: 63, www.biomed central.com/1741-7015/11/63.

7 J.E. Lee et al. (2013), 'Meat intake and cause-specific mortality: a pooled analysis of Asian prospective cohort studies', *Am J Clin Nutr* 98: 1032–41.

8 Reported by G. Gustin (23 March 2016), 'Another nation trims meat from diet advice', *National Geographic*, http://theplate.nationalgeo graphic.com/2016/03/23/nother-nation-trims-meat-from-diet-advice.

9 R.A. Koeth et al. (2013), 'Intestinal microbiota metabolism of

L-carnitine, a nutrient in red meat, promotes atherosclerosis', *Nature Medicine* 19: 576–85.

10 en.m.wikipedia.org/wiki/'Red_meat'. Accessed 23 December 2015.

11 Harvard School of Public Health (2011), *Healthy Eating Plate and Healthy Eating Pyramid*, www.hsph.harvard.edu/nutritionsource/ healthy-eating-plate/. Accessed 23 December 2015.

12 G.K. Pot et al. (2010), 'Increased consumption of fatty and lean fish reduces serum C-Reactive Protein concentrations but not inflammation markers in feces and in colonic biopsies', *J Nutr* 140: 371–6.

13 H.O. Bang and J. Dyerberg (5 June 1971), 'Plasma lipid and lipoprotein pattern in Greenlandic west-coast Eskimos', *Lancet* 297: 1143–6.

14 J.H. Lett et al. (2008), 'Omega-3 fatty acids for cardioprotection', *Mayo Clin Proc* 83: 324–32.

15 G.K. Pot et al. (2010), 'Increased consumption of fatty and lean fish reduces serum C-Reactive Protein concentrations but not inflammation markers in feces and in colonic biopsies', *J Nutr* 140: 371–6.

16 Reported by G. Gustin (23 March 2016), 'Another nation trims meat from diet advice', *National Geographic*, http://theplate.nationalgeo graphic.com/2016/03/23/another-nation-trims-meat-from-diet-advice.

17 J.C. Ratliff et al. (2008), 'Eggs modulate the inflammatory response to carbohydrate restricted diets in overweight men', *Nutr Metabol* 5: 6, doi:10.1186/1743-7075-5-6.

18 J.K. Virtanen et al. (2015), 'Egg consumption and incident type 2 diabetes in men: the Kuopio Ischaemic Heart Disease Risk Factor Study', *Am J Clin Nutr*, doi: 10.3945/ajcn.114.104109.

19 J.W. Krieger et al. (2006), 'Effect of variation in protein and carbohydrate intake on body mass and composition during energy restriction: a meta-regression', *Am J Clin Nutr* 83: 260–74.

20 P. Lymberry and I. Oakshott (2014), *Farmageddon: The True Cost of Cheap Meat*, Bloomsbury, London.

21 U. Ericson et al. (2015), 'Food sources of fat may clarify the inconsistent role of dietary fat intake for incidence of type 2 diabetes', *Am J Clin Nutr* 101, doi: 10.3945/ajcn.114.103010.

22 M.-E. Labonte et al. (2013), 'Impact of dairy products on biomarkers of inflammation: a systematic review of randomized controlled nutritional intervention studies in overweight and obese adults', *Am J Clin Nutr* 87: 706–17.

23 H. Hjerpsted et al. (2011), 'Cheese intake in large amounts lowers LDL-cholesterol concentrations compared with butter intake of equal fat content', *Am J Clin Nutr* 94: 1479–84.

24 D.J.A. Jenkins et al. (2014), 'Effect of a 6-month vegan low-carbohydrate ("Eco-Atkins") diet on cardiovascular risk factors and body weight in hyperlipidaemic adults: a randomised controlled trial', *BMJ Open* 4: e003505.

25 Joe Leech (March 2015), 'What is the healthiest oil for deep frying? The crispy truth', *Authority Nutrition*, Authoritynutrition.com/healthiestoil-fordeep-frying. Accessed December 2015.

26 A. Pan et al. (2013), 'Walnut consumption is associated with lower risk of type 2 diabetes in women', *J Nutr* 143: 512–18.

27 P. Wurtz et al. (2015), 'Metabolite profiling and cardiovascular event risk: a prospective study of three population-based cohorts', *Circulation* 131: 774–85.

28 S. Basu et al. (2013), 'The relationship of sugar to population-level diabetes prevalence: an econometric analysis of repeated cross-sectional data', *PLOS ONE* 8: e57873. Doi:10.1371/journal.pone. 0057873.

29 P. Bee (20 April 2015), 'The end of fruit?', *The Times* 2: 6–7.

30 A.M. Stephens and J.H. Cummings (1980), 'The microbial contribution to human faecal fat mass', *J Med Microbiol* 13: 45–56.

31 F. Backhed et al. (2007), 'Mechanisms underlying the resistance to diet-induced obesity in germ-free mice', *PNAS* 104: 979–84.

32 O. Koren et al. (2012), 'Host remodelling of the gut microbiome and metabolic changes during pregnancy', *Cell* 150: 470–80.

33 H. Hjerpsted et al. (2011), 'Cheese intake in large amounts lowers LDL-cholesterol concentrations compared with butter intake of equal fat content', *Am J Clin Nutr* 94: 1478–84.

34 B. Chassaing et al. (2015), 'Dietary emulsifiers impact the mouse gut microbiota promoting colitis and metabolic syndrome', *Nature* 519: 92–6.

35 M. Pollan (2009), *Food Rules: An Eater's Manual*, Penguin Press, New York.

36 R. Lustig (2013), *Fat Chance*, Hudson Street Press, New York, p. 172.

29: And if you must eat breakfast?

1 K. Foster-Powell et al. (2002), 'International table of glycemic index and glycemic load values: 2002', *Am J Clin Nutr* 76: 5–56.

2 http://care.diabetesjournals.org/content/suppl/2008/09/18/dc08-1239.DC1/TableA1_1.pdf.

3 Harvard Medical School (27 August 2015), 'Glycemic index and glycemic load for 100+ foods', www.health.harvard.edu/healthy-eating/glycemic_index_and_glycemic_load_for_100_foods. Accessed 8 April 2016.

4 *Diabetes Care* (2015), 38: Supplement, S1–93, 'Standards of medical care in diabetes – 2015'. © 2105 by the American Diabetes Association. http://care.diabetesjournals.org/content/suppl/2014/12/23/38.Supplement_1.DC1/January_Supplement_Combined_Final.6-99.pdf.

5 A.R. Last et al. (2006), 'Low-carbohydrate diets', *Am Fam Phys*, http://www.aafp.org/afp/2006/0601/p1942.htmol. Accessed 8 August 2016.

6 M.J. Chen et al. (2010), 'Utilizing the second-meal effect in type 2 diabetes: practical use of a soya-yogurt snack', *Diabetes Care* 33: 2552–4.

7 A. Frustaci et al. (1997), 'Histological substrate of atrial biopsies in patients with lone atrial fibrillation', *Circulation* 96: 1180–84.

8 Mayo Clinic (9 December 2011), *Alcohol and Diabetes: Drinking Safely*, www.mayoclinic.org/diseases-conditions/diabetes/expert-blog/alcohol-and-diabetes/bgp-20056464.

9 Diabetes UK (2016), *Alcohol*, www.diabetes.org.uk/Guide-to-diabetes/Managing-your-diabetes/Alcohol/. Accessed 31 March 2016.

Envoi

1 Sarah Churchill (1981), *Keep on Dancing*, Weidenfeld and Nicolson, London, p. 18.

Afterword

1 H.-J. Chen et al. (2016), 'Relationship between frequency of eating and cardiovascular disease in US adults: the NHANES III follow-up study', *Ann Epidemiol*, http://dx.doi.org/10.1016/j.annepidem.2016.06.006.

2 M.G. Marmot et al. (1997), 'Contribution of job control and other risk factors to social variations in heart disease incidence', *Lancet* 350: 235–9.

Illustration credits

Figure 1.1 From Guido Freckmann, et al. (2007), 'Continuous glucose profiles in healthy subjects under everyday life conditions and after different meals', *J Diabetes Sci Technol* 1: 695–703.

Figure 1.2a From T. Parkner, et al. (2011), 'Do all patients with type 2 diabetes need breakfast?', *Eur J Clin Nutr* 65: 761–3.

Figure 1.2b Ibid.

Figure 17.1 From K.S. Polonsky, et al. (1988), 'Twenty-four-hour profiles and pulsatile patterns of insulin secretion in normal and obese subjects', *J Clin Invest* 81: 442–8.

Figure 18.1 From S.-S. Zhou, et al. (2010), 'B-vitamin consumption and the prevalence of diabetes and obesity among US adults: population based ecological study', *BMC Public Health* 10: 746.

Figure 21.1 From B. Selamaoui and Y. Touitou (2003), 'Reproducibility of the circadian rhythm of serum cortisol and melatonin in healthy subjects: a study of three different 24-h cycles of six weeks', *Life Sci* 73: 3339–49.

Figure 21.2 From L. Stryer (1995), *Biochemistry* (fourth edition), W.H. Freeman and Company, New York, pp. 603–28.

Figure 24.1 From B. Lewis (1973), 'Classification of lipoproteins and lipoprotein disorders', *J Clin Pathol* S5: 26–31.

Acknowledgements

Challenging the consensus on breakfast has not always been easy, and I might never have completed this project but for the help of my friends. My first thanks go to the medical and nursing staff at the Swan Practice in Buckingham, who not only looked after me so well but who also inspired this book by providing me with a glucometer (or glucose meter) that, to my surprise, revealed that breakfast was for me a dangerous meal.

Second, I thank my good friend the late Professor Mike Cawthorne, the professor of biochemistry at the University of Buckingham, who told me that 'everything the NHS, NICE [the National Institute for Health and Care Excellence] and the diabetes charities say about carbohydrates is of course wrong'. I also thank Julie Cakebread and Eddie Shoesmith of the University for their scientific input into this book. My other friends at Buckingham are legion, but sadly they work within non-breakfast-relevant disciplines, so I cannot name them here.

Third, I thank Professor Sir Christopher Edwards FMedSci, whose houseman I was back in 1976, who told me of other discoveries that contradicted NICE's guidelines and who encouraged me to be sceptical of official advice.

Fourth, I thank my old friend Professor Roy Taylor of Newcastle University, who has long seen through the breakfast propaganda and who was kind enough to read some of the chapters of this book at an early stage. Any mistakes that have survived are of course solely mine, but thanks to Roy there are fewer of them.

Three people who have always supported my science writing are Matt Ridley, Nassim Taleb and Professor David Edgerton of King's College London, and I'm happy to thank them here. I have, moreover, breakfast-insightful friends at the Cato Institute in Washington, DC, with whom I spent most of 2016, and I thank Roshni Ashar, Chip Knappenberger, Pat Michaels, Guillermina Sutter and Joe Verruni for all their help.

My wife, Sally, has been my best support; she's read draft chapters and spotted interesting articles in the newspapers, and I'm so happy not only to thank her but also to dedicate this book to her. I also thank Helena and Teddy, our children, for tolerating my lectures over their breakfasts and sugary indulgences.

This book was hugely improved by Louise Haines from 4th Estate, and I thank her, David Roth-Ey (who is very sound on breakfast) and Sarah Thickett for all that they did: they were great. I also thank Jamie Keenan for a terrific cover and Felicity Bryan for being a superb agent.

Index